Toward a Theory for Nursing

WILEY PAPERBACK NURSING SERIES

Toward a Theory for Nursing

GENERAL CONCEPTS OF HUMAN BEHAVIOR

Imogene M. King, R.N., Ed.D.

Director, School of Nursing
The Ohio State University
Columbus, Ohio

JOHN WILEY AND SONS, INC.

New York / London / Sydney / Toronto

Library of Congress Catalogue Card Number: 70-136716

ISBN 0-471-47800-8

Printed in the United States of America

10 9 8 7

This book is dedicated to my Sister
for her support, encouragement
and kindness over the years.

Wiley Paperback Nursing Series

This unique series provides the nursing profession with current and timely information. The five volumes do not follow a single theme. Some volumes deal with topics that are particularly interesting to undergraduate and graduate college students, some deal with matters that appeal to nursing educators, and others consider problems that confront practicing nurses and persons in the nursing service.

Many of these books are appropriate for use in both graduate and undergraduate courses. The contributors have selected their subjects with care. Each author possesses the interest, background, and experience necessary to deal comprehensively with the chosen subject.

Ever-expanding general knowledge and the rapid advances in the medical and health fields make it imperative that nurses have readily available materials that are relevant to their needs. I believe this series accomplishes this purpose and that it is an important contribution to the nursing profession.

Nurses, teachers, and students alike should find these books helpful and stimulating.

MILDRED MONTAG
Teachers' College,
Columbia University

Preface

Nursing is in a period of transition. Social and educational changes in the United States in the past few decades have influenced nursing directly and indirectly. Advancements in science and technology have caused changes in environmental conditions, in prevalence and incidence of disease, and in preventive and curative means available for use by health professionals.

The scientific foundations of nursing practice have been challenged by some nurses, especially in the past decade. Some nurses claim that today, more than ever before, decision making by professional nurses must be based on an organized body of knowledge selected for its relevance to nursing practice. It has been said that the nurse's involvement at every level of society is essential for the delivery of health services. However, several studies of the nurse's role have indicated that changes have brought about conflict and controversy relative to the nurse's values.

The purpose of this book is to propose a conceptual frame of reference for nursing. It is intended to be utilized specifically by students and teachers, and also by researchers and practitioners to identify and analyze events in specific nursing situations. The framework suggests that the essential characteristics of nursing are those properties that have persisted in spite of environmental changes. A concept of health, which I perceive to include illness and alterations in health states, is discussed in relation to nursing.

A personal concern about the changes influencing nursing, a conscious awareness of the knowledge explosion, and a hunch that some of the essential components of nursing have persisted, prompted the exploration of several questions. What are some of the social and educational changes in the United States that have influenced changes in nursing? What basic elements are continuous throughout these changes in nursing? What is the scope of the practice of nursing, and in what kind of settings do nurses perform their functions? Are the current goals of nursing similar to those of the past half century? What are the dimensions of practice that have given the field of nursing a unifying focus over time?

Responses to these questions have led to the selection of four universal ideas—social systems, health, perception, and interpersonal relations—and to an exploration of their relevance to nursing. These ideas provide a general frame of reference for identifying concepts that suggest more specific directives for nursing practice.

The plan of the book is to discuss in Chapter 1 approaches suggested by some nurses to develop theoretical frames of reference for nursing. In Chapter 2 the need for formulating conceptual frames of reference for nursing is presented. Chapter 3 suggests uses for the framework presented in this book for teaching, for practicing, and for studying nursing. Chapter 4 presents a *concept of social systems* as one dimension of nursing. The goal of nursing—*health*—is suggested in Chapter 5 and Chapter 6 offers a description of the dynamics of nursing practice—*perception* and *interpersonal relations*. Chapter 7 indicates some of the factors that have influenced changes in nursing. The last chapter summarizes the main points of the book.

The sources used by the author are selective rather than comprehensive. There are multiple studies and reports available relative to each idea. It is hoped that this volume will generate ideas for students, teachers, practitioners, administrators, and researchers to assist them in formulating their own conceptual frame of reference for nursing. It should prompt employers and other professionals to react, to interact, and to collaborate with nurses to improve the delivery of health services to the public.

Imogene M. King

April, 1970

Acknowledgments

This book represents a synthesis of the ideas of many individuals. I express my gratitude and thanks to all the persons who listened to me, who shared ideas with me, and who raised critical questions about my own ideas. It is not possible to mention all of the individuals by name.

However, I am greatly indebted to Dr. Hildgard E. Peplau and Dr. Mildred L. Montag for reasons they alone will understand. Finally, I want to express my appreciation to the publishers and journals who have granted permission to use copyrighted material.

I.M.K.

Contents

Toward a Theory for Nursing

Chapter 1

Introduction

Nursing is part of many social systems; it arises from and functions within social systems. Nursing is changed by and alters itself in response to constantly changing social forces within a culture; it also influences changes in society and its institutions. Nursing finds its heritage deeply rooted in the past, its transition in the present, and its future unpredictable. The roles and responsibilities of nurses are multidimensional and involve both individuals and groups in social systems. Nursing practice at its best is based on an understanding of man, from conception to old age, in health and in illness.

For example, knowledge of the family as a social system is important in assisting individuals to meet their basic human needs. An understanding of how the family and other social systems in the environment impinge on health, positively or negatively, is an essential facet in the nurse's armamentarium. Hence, it is imperative that new relationships between the scientific discoveries in other fields of study and in nursing are identified and utilized.

The vast expansion of knowledge and increased specialization, especially within the health professions, have created several problems. One of these problems is the need to identify the essential components of nursing practice that persist despite the diverse educational programs, the new technologies, and the numerous pieces of health legislation passed by Congress in the past few years.

A primary concern of this book is to explore dimensions of nursing and to propose a conceptual frame of reference for professional nursing. Facts that continue to accumulate from new discoveries are too numerous to teach and to learn in a formal educational program. Facts if not used are soon forgotten. A framework provides an efficient and economical way of organizing knowledge. Teachers are being challenged to identify and select relevant concepts that can be developed with nursing students. These concepts require a focus—a framework of essentials —central to the field of nursing practice.

This book has departed from previous attempts by nurses to formulate theoretical approaches for nursing. It sorts out of the social and educational changes those elements that continue to represent the foundations for nursing practice, and offers suggestions for a reorientation to the goal of nursing.

Research in nursing has only recently begun to explore the nature of nursing practice. A review of nursing research in the past decade indicates that theoretical formulations for nursing practice are limited. The findings from nursing research at this time are not yet adequate for making generalizations or predictions about nursing practice. Analysis of nursing research, however, gives us clues about basic concepts relevant for nursing practice. These clues have been very useful in view of the purpose of this book, which is to make explicit a conceptual frame of reference for nursing, and to indicate an approach for organizing knowledge for learning the practice of professional nursing.

Previous Efforts to Provide a Framework

In the past two decades a number of authors have suggested ways of organizing a knowledge base relevant to nursing practice. The most recent work by Martha Rogers[1] offers a theoretical basis for nursing. Four reports of a study conducted under the auspices of

[1] Martha E. Rogers, *An Introduction to the Theoretical Basis for Nursing,* F. A. Davis Co., Philadelphia, 1970.

the Western Council on Higher Education for Nursing, [2,3,4,5] demonstrated the first regional group efforts to organize knowledge by defining "clinical content for graduate programs" in nursing. A different frame of reference was proposed by each of the four groups of nurse faculty members in higher education in Community Health Nursing, Medical-Surgical Nursing, Maternal-Child Health Nursing, and Psychiatric Mental Health Nursing. Each group noted, either explicitly or implicitly, that nursing content is a synthesis of principles, concepts, laws, and theories from the natural and social sciences. Each group discussed concepts perceived as relevant for each specialized field of nursing. Analysis of the reports indicates that basic human needs of individuals were deemed important by each group. A detailed analysis of these documents may provide clues for a theoretical frame of reference for general nursing practice.

Quint[6] calls attention to observations in the real world as a tool for studying patient care. She notes that the problem to be studied can be designed for the purpose of determining a conceptual frame of reference for events in nursing situations rather than of testing hypotheses from a predetermined formal theory.

One example of the use of existing theories was discussed by Cleland[7] at a symposium on research in nursing in 1966. She noted that nurses can abstract meaningful concepts from theoretical formulations from reported research and then express the empirical problem to be studied. Cleland stated clearly the usefulness of theory: selecting a nursing problem "permits the researcher to use theory as a functional method by which to work deductively from theoretical formulations and inductively from existing empirical data."

2 The Western Council on Higher Education for Nursing (WCHEN), Defining Clinical Content, Graduate Nursing Programs, *Maternal-Child Health Nursing*, Western Interstate Commission for Higher Education (WICHE), Boulder, Colorado, 1967.

3 WCHEN, *Psychiatric Nursing*, WICHE, Boulder, Colorado, 1967.

4 WCHEN, *Community Health Nursing*, WICHE, Boulder, Colorado, 1967.

5 WCHEN, *Medical-Surgical Nursing*, WICHE, Boulder, Colorado, 1967.

6 Jeanne Quint, "The Case for Theories Generated from Empirical Data," *Nursing Research*, Spring 1967, pp. 109-114.

7 Virginia S. Cleland, "The Use of Existing Theories," *Nursing Research*, Spring 1967, pp. 118-121.

A plea for basic research in nursing is made by Rogers: "the application of knowledge depends on the unifying principles and hypothetical generalizations growing out of basic research in nursing."[8] Her fundamental postulates about man and his relationship with the universe represent a rationale for viewing man as a dynamic organism moving on a continuum of life from minimum to maximum states of well-being.[9] Her concept of man and his relationship to the universe gives nursing one of its principal reasons for existing, and for pursuing basic research.

Brown[10] has reinforced the ideas of other nurses and notes that nurse investigators must meet the challenge of building theory by making explicit their theoretical framework and the way the research will build a body of knowledge for nursing.

Ways in which some of the theories from biological and behavioral sciences can help nurses identify and study nursing problems are described by Gunter.[11] She suggests that a "theory of the organism, a theory of medicine, and a theory of interpersonal relations in combination" may provide a framework whereby nursing functions can be distinguished from those of medical and paramedical groups.

Peplau's[12] conceptual frame of reference demonstrated the usefulness of interpersonal theories such as those of Sullivan, Fromm, and others. She defines the nature of nursing and its relationship to human life and health in terms of interpersonal relations. She gives nurses a body of concepts about interpersonal relationships focused on selected examples collected through direct observations in various types of nursing situations.

In the preface of Orlando's[13] book, her stated purpose is to

[8] Martha E. Rogers, *Reveille in Nursing,* F. A. Davis Co., Philadelphia, 1964, p. 10.

[9] Martha E. Rogers, *Educational Revolution in Nursing,* Macmillan, New York, 1961, pp. 16-22.

[10] M. Irene Brown, "Research in the Development of Nursing Theory," *Nursing Research,* Spring 1964, p. 110.

[11] Laurie M. Gunter, "Notes on a Theoretical Framework for Nursing," *Nursing Research,* Fall 1962, pp. 219-222.

[12] Hildegard E. Peplau, *Interpersonal Relations in Nursing,* G. P. Putnam's Sons, New York, 1952.

[13] Ida Jean Orlando, *The Dynamic Nurse-Patient Relationship,* G. P. Putnam's Sons, New York, 1961, p. viii.

"offer the professional nursing student a theory of effective nursing practice." Function, process, and principles of professional nursing practice are identified through analysis of elements in nursing situations. The theme of the book revolves around the use of a deliberative nursing process in analyzing the problems of patients and in the effectiveness of the nurse in helping patients resolve problems and achieve goals.

Brown and Fowler[14] agree with Peplau and Orlando in the conceptualization of nursing as a process of interaction. They discuss a conceptual frame of reference and state that it is a "somewhat embryonic theory of nursing." They relate the nursing process to significant dimensions of the social system and the range of interaction of the recipient of nursing care. Some of the resources identified in the social system are persons, events, objects, and the basic needs of individuals related to activities of daily living.

A recent study of older individuals in specified institutional settings has provided a conceptual model to describe nurse-patient interaction. The concepts in the model relate to psychosocial systems, dimensions, processes, and resources in the systems, and the development or changes in the systems.[15]

Some nurses have attempted to identify principles from the natural and social sciences and to demonstrate their use in nursing situations. This was the approach of Nordmark and Rohweder's[16] initial study of scientific principles, that has been expanded in their recent publication.[17]

Another means used to systematize the knowledge base for practice is the classification of nursing problems, such as the typology of Abdellah, et al.[18] These ideas are expanded by Matheney and

14 Martha M. Brown and Grace R. Fowler, *Psychodynamic Nursing: A Bio-Social Orientation*, W. B. Saunders Co., Philadelphia, 1966, pp. 123-124.

15 James M. A. Weiss (ed.), *Nurses, Patients, and Social Systems*, University of Missouri Press, Columbia, Mo., 1968, p. 6.

16 Madelyn T. Nordmark and Anne W. Rohweder, *Science Principles Applied to Nursing*, J. B. Lippincott, Philadelphia, 1959.

17 Madelyn T. Nordmark and Anne W. Rohweder, *Scientific Foundations of Nursing*, J. B. Lippincott, Philadelphia, 1967.

18 Faye G. Abdellah, Irene L. Beland, Almeda Martin, Ruth V. Matheney, *Patient Centered Approaches to Nursing*, Macmillan, New York, 1961.

others as fundamental knowledge essential for the practice of nursing.[19]

McCain's[20] concept of nursing "incorporates the belief that the primary goal of nursing care is to assist a patient attain and maintain a state of equilibrium as he reacts to internal and external stimuli." She proposes a method for systematic assessment of nursing needs of patients. The method of assessment includes specific functional abilities of patients within four major categories: mental status, emotional status, sensory perception, and motor ability. McCain notes that a precise method of collecting information about the physiologic, psychologic, and social behavior of patient provides a rationale for planning, guiding, and evaluating nursing care.

Social forces, especially the past decade, have influenced changes in nursing. Some of these forces are relevant to the direct and personal service called nursing care identified and discussed by Johnson.[21] She notes that the functional abilities of individuals and groups tend to be constant and stabilized in health, and that "stabilized and constant patterns of functioning are possible and even necessary in illness." She discusses the stability-constancy concept using the terms equilibrium, stress, and tension. She notes, too, that the primary objectives of nursing care deal with immediate situations and that universal human needs are the focus for nursing activities.

Kaufmann's[22] approach to identify a theoretical basis for nursing practice resulted in the construction of a model based on concepts of time, perception, and stress and their relationship to nursing. She considers the model as one of "motion and ongoingness" and perception as the "energizing dimension of the model." Time is

[19] Ruth V. Matheney, Breda T. Nolan, Alice M. Ehrhart, Gerald J. Griffin, Joanne K. Griffin, *Fundamentals of Patient Centered Nursing*, The C. V. Mosby Co., St. Louis, Mo., 1964.

[20] Faye McCain, "Nursing By Assessment—Not By Intuition," *American Journal of Nursing*, April 1965, pp. 82-84.

[21] Dorothy E. Johnson, "The Significance of Nursing Care," *American Journal of Nursing*, November 1961, pp. 63-66.

[22] Margaret Anne Kaufmann, *Identification of Theoretical Bases for Nursing Practice*, unpublished doctoral dissertation, University of California, Los Angeles, 1958.

an element that is viewed in the present, influenced by the past, and projected to the future. Culture, experience, and learning are major inputs in the model; these are broad dimensions of the life process with which nurses deal. Within the model, stress is considered the largest input contributor by volume, but perception is of greatest importance since it controls the quantity and types of stress that enter the perceptual field. This generic theoretical model provides nurses with a basis for theory development. It provides a framework for describing nursing situations and for generating hypotheses to test in nursing situations.

The organization of a body of knowledge for nursing is, in the opinion of the author, a major problem facing the profession. Reports in the nursing literature indicate a need for identifying theories that are relevant for nursing. Why this emphasis on theory development in nursing at this point in the history of the profession? There are probably many reasons, one of which is the vast accumulation of knowledge from research. Another reason is the number of nurses with advanced degrees who are asking questions about nursing as a discipline. Yet another reason is the fact that a discipline in higher education is expected to have a theoretical body of knowledge that can be taught and learned; in a practice discipline the knowledge is applied by the practitioner. Still another reason is the fact that the action research in associate degree nursing programs demonstrated technical education for nursing. It is essential now to make explicit the scientific foundations for professional education for nursing to differentiate between professional nursing practice and technical and vocational practice of nursing. The differentiation of levels of nursing practice on the basis of levels of education will continue to be a problem in the health field until concepts are made explicit resulting in a professional language in nursing that will enhance communication and understanding at all levels of practice. One approach to this problem is to increase descriptive and explanatory research into nursing practice that will help nurses visualize and articulate phenomena in a system of relations—a framework.

Summary

The purpose of this book is to synthesize some of the thinking, the research, and the writing of nurses and individuals in related fields toward a general theory for nursing. If nurses are to continue to search for and to explicate the scientific foundations for nursing practice, theoretical formulations are essential. The building blocks of theories are concepts. The concepts identified by many nurses cited here indicate a movement in nursing to identify and test theories for nursing.

Selected Readings

Berelson, Bernard, and Steiner, Gary, *Human Behavior*, Harcourt Brace, New York, 1964.

Berthold, Jeanne, "Theoretical and Empirical Clarification of Concepts," *Nursing Science*, October 1964, pp. 406-422.

Daedalus, "Theory in Humanistic Studies," *Journal of the American Academy of Arts and Sciences*, Spring 1970.

Hadley, Betty Jo, "Evolution of a Conception of Nursing," *Nursing Research*, September-October 1969, pp. 400-404.

Johnson, Dorothy E., "The Nature of a Science of Nursing," *Nursing Outlook*, May 1959, pp. 291-294.

King, Imogene M., "Nursing Theory—Problems and Prospect," *Nursing Science*, October 1964, pp. 394-403.

McKay, Rose, "Theories, Models, and Systems for Nursing," *Nursing Research*, September-October 1969, pp. 393-399.

Smith, Martha R., "A Concept of Nursing," *American Journal of Nursing*, June 1933, p. 565.

Taylor, Effie, "Of What Is the Nature of Nursing," *American Journal of Nursing*, May 1934, p. 476.

Chapter 2

A Conceptual Frame of Reference for Nursing

The changes in society, the various types of educational programs that prepare nurses for diverse occupations, the information explosion, and the increasing demands for specialization have pointed to a need for some unifying focus for nursing. History shows that nursing has been an applied science; that is, it has used knowledge from a variety of sources and in a practical way. This pattern of borrowing knowledge from natural and social sciences has been followed in the birth of most fields of study. In a field whose purpose is to provide a social service to meet a social need, the generation and dissemination of knowledge is incomplete if theory is not related to practice. Research and graduate education are inseparable components of this idea that professional nursing practice has its foundations grounded in theories that are continuously subjected to testing and validation in the real world.

Need for Conceptual Frameworks for Nursing

Communication between nurse practitioners, teachers, administrators, and researchers is often impeded by the language used. Ways of communicating changes in the profession and of disseminating new knowledge is essential to guard against further disarticulation between these groups. As a step toward resolving some of the communication problems, we may begin by identifying concepts that are useful for nurses. A common understanding of the concepts being developed with nursing students as learners and those used in the practice of nursing in real situations will help graduates in their transition from the role of learner to the role of practitioner.

Teachers and practitioners are faced with increasingly complex problems. One major problem is the increase in quantity of scientific facts and new technology. In view of the increasing amount and complexity of information and theories in all fields, it is incumbent upon teachers of nursing to guide students in learning ways of thinking, methods of studying, ways of selecting basic information, and of applying knowledge in order to begin to function as practitioners. If students develop fundamental concepts as learners, then as practitioners their conceptual frame of reference will accommodate new knowledge throughout the continuous life-long process of learning.

New knowledge may also influence nurses to change their frame of reference over time. Moreover, concepts offer an approach to understanding interacting systems and the relationship of individuals and groups in any environment. Methodology does not yet exist to deal with the complexity of nursing situations. Nurses have been introduced to knowledge from natural and behavioral sciences, and have been expected to synthesize this knowledge for use in nursing practice. *Generally, the basic abstraction of nursing is the phenomenon of man and his world.* One approach to working within such complexity is to identify specific goals for nursing care to determine ways that individuals and groups cope with health and illness and adapt to changes in health states. One of the means used by some individuals is the identification of concepts.

What Are Concepts?

In the process of knowing, a person gains an impression of an object by the use of the senses. Concepts are mental images formed by generalizations from these particular impressions. A construct, in turn, is a group of related ideas (concepts) descriptive of the real world. When behaviors, characteristics, or actions are identified and operationally defined these elements of a concept can be measured.

Concepts are abstract ideas that give meaning to our sense perceptions, permit generalizations, and tend to be stored in our memory for recall and use at a later time in new and different situations. Initially, we may think of concepts as word symbols; this approach has been used in this book.

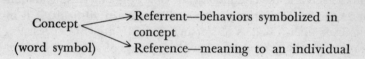

Some words, such as government, health, stress, man, culture, in a common language deal with concepts—universal terms that characterize properties and relations of a class of things, persons, objects. Word explication is one method of discovering underlying concepts. Words provide a means of organizing ideas, and these in turn bring order to disconnected observations, related experiences, and effect economy of thought.

Perception is the process by which senses transmit meaning to the brain; these acts of perception help formulate concepts which give meaning to life for each individual. Each person develops his own concepts and this is done through directly perceiving a thing, object, person, or event. A concept is not a concrete entity in nature; it is each individual's abstraction of the real world.

Concepts, then, provide individuals with symbolic representations, and a description of characteristics or attributes of objects and events in nursing situations. A basic vocabulary of words with which nurses can communicate with each other about persons, objects, and events in their universe is essential in developing a scientific foundation for nursing.

What is Theory?

In the past, the content of nursing courses has been widely identified as "nursing theory" to differentiate the formal classroom teaching from the practice in the laboratory. Such theory often consisted of taxonomies of disease, biological systems, medical categories, and practical techniques. However, this application of the term "theory" has, at times, precluded using the word in its broader, more scientific sense.

One idea common to many writers is that theory is the identification of concepts which, when defined, correspond to observable phenomena and are interrelated. Merton, for example, noted:

Concepts, then, constitute the definitions of what is to be observed; they are the variables between which empirical relationships are to be sought. When propositions are logically interrelated, a theory has been instituted.[1]

A description of the basic terms of a theory indicates that the concepts have a relationship to observable phenomena and to other terms in the theory. The concepts of one science or theory may become the basic terms of another science or theory.

Theory has been described as a game with words. Words are symbols of man's view of his world. No matter what level of theory is being constructed in a field of study, it must have some way of getting down to the raw materials of objects, persons, and events in the everyday world. One rule in theory building, therefore, is that the meaning of the terms clearly describe phenomena in the real world.

Nagel's[2] analysis of the cognitive status of theories indicates that three components can usually be isolated in a theory, namely, "an abstract set of postulates which implicitly define the basic terms of the theory, a model or interpretation for the postulates, and rules of correspondence for terms in the postulates or in the theorems derived from them." In his discussion of the instrumentalists' ideas of theory, he states:

Theories are intellectual tools, not physical ones. They are nevertheless conceptual frameworks deliberately devised for effectively directing experimental inquiry and for exhibiting connections between matters of observation that would otherwise be regarded as unrelated.[3]

[1] Robert Merton, *Social Theory and Social Structure*, Macmillan, New York, 1957, p. 55.
[2] Ernest Nagel, *The Structure of Science*, Harcourt Brace and World, New York, 1961, p. 106.
[3] Ibid., p. 131.

Specific formulas for building theory are difficult to find. Homans,[4] however, enunciates the following general rules:

1. Look first at the obvious, the familiar, the common. In a science that has not established its foundations, these are the things that best repay study.
2. State the obvious in its full generality. Science is an economy of thought only if its hypotheses add up in a simple form a large number of facts.
3. Talk about one thing at a time. That is, in choosing your words (or, more pedantically, concepts) see that they refer not to several classes of fact at the same time but to one and only one. Corollary: once you have chosen your words always use the same words when referring to the same thing.
4. Cut down as far as you dare the number of things you are talking about. As few as you may; as many as you must is the rule governing the number of classes between the facts designated by your words.
5. Once you have started to talk, do not stop until you have finished. That is, describe systematically the relationships between the facts designated by your words.
6. Recognize that your analysis must be abstract, because it deals with only a few elements of the concrete situation. Admit the danger of abstractions, especially when action is required, but do not be afraid of abstractions.

In writing about a unified theory of behavior, Grinker[5] notes that "what we need is first approximation to a scheme which will enable us to represent physical, psychological and social events within one system of denotation." If such a model could be formulated, it would stimulate an entirely new approach to studying the complex relations between the body, mind, and socioeconomic events. A framework would result in which the individual and his surroundings, both in health and illness, would be considered simultaneously.

If nursing is a science, then nurses must be aware of the characteristics of science that provide the means to develop a systematic body of knowledge for nursing. These characteristics are

4 George C. Homans, *The Human Group*, Harcourt Brace, New York, 1950, pp. 16-17.
5 Roy R. Grinker (ed.), *Toward a Unified Theory of Human Behavior*, Basic Books, New York, 1965, p. xi.

certainty (if A, then B will follow), *structure,* which indicates relationships, and *generalizations,* which are derived from research findings. These characteristics of scientific knowledge provide nurses with a means to assess the scientific basis of nursing and continue to develop a systematic body of knowledge for nursing. These phases for identifying scientific knowledge are: (1) description, (2) explanation, (3) prediction. In a practice discipline predictions provide a basis for prescribing action in specific situations. If nursing is a science, then the body of knowledge taught, learned, and used by professional nurses is characterized by certainty, structure, and generalizations. If nursing is a profession, then scientific knowledge forms the foundations for learning the practice of the profession. Have you been able to find in nursing literature any theories that form the basis for professional practice? Nursing as a young field in research has moved rapidly in the past decade to identify some of the major issues and problems facing the profession. Research into the nature of nursing practice is a primary problem. When a body of scientific knowledge is developed for nursing, then nurses can understand theories that form the basis for professional practice.

What Are the Sources of Theory?

Practitioners, teachers, administrators and researchers are a few of the sources of theory. Adaptation of theoretical models from other disciplines is another source of theory. Theories may be discovered in the real world of nursing practice through systematic collection of data about specific phenomena. The current practitioners have some ideas about phenomena that consistently occur in nursing situations. A staff nurse in a neurological unit in a large hospital was asked if she observed any consistent patterns of patient behavior and response in pre- and postoperative patients who had similar pathology (brain tumor). She noted that each one of the three patients responded in similar patterns postoperatively. She has wondered about these phenomena she continues to observe in her practice and would like to find some answers to her hunches. Three nurses in coronary care units in three different regions of the country, South, Midwest, and West, mentioned they had observed that patients could not recall events in their hospitalization immediately following a crisis. Some practitioners in the course of their observations see similar patterns of behavioral responses, yet lack of time and of knowledge of the research process does not permit them to systematically record their observations for analysis to discover common patterns of behavior of individuals in stressful situations.

Analysis of research findings in nursing literature and related fields may lead to some speculation, to hypotheses testing, and to theory development. Selecting the postulates or propositions of a theory in another discipline and testing them in nursing situations is another source of theory. Role deprivation, for example, or social deprivation are concepts from social psychology that have relevance for nursing. Analysis of concepts that appear to be fundamental to nursing practice, that are discussed by nurses, and appear in nursing literature, are yet another source for theory. Theories can originate within the field of nursing or can be borrowed from another field and tested in nursing through research. You may be asking yourself at this moment, "What will all of this theorizing do for patient care, for health care, for nursing? Is it not just an intellectual exercise? Is it a status seeking kind of activity?" If theory is not useful, it really is not worth the effort to develop it.

Usefulness of Theory for Nurses and Nursing

Theory provides a way to organize a multitude of facts into more meaningful wholes. Theory gives an organized, efficient, and economical way of learning and practicing nursing, and gives some idea of the consequences of nursing action. Theory provides a starting point for systematic collection of facts to describe and explain nursing situations and can extend the range of nursing knowledge. Theory provides a communication system in terms of a set of concepts that are interrelated and understandable to others. Theory provides a set of interrelated hypotheses that may make predications about empirical events, and offer prescriptions for nursing action. Theories direct attention to processes and relationships relevant for nursing practice. Ways to order knowledge in a variety of nursing situations are provided by theories.

How will the recipient of nursing care and the profession benefit from these activities in which theories are developed and continuously tested in nursing practice? Theories would be helpful in several ways: (1) nurses would be in a position to judge or test the effectiveness of their practice; if theories were unacceptable, practice would be unacceptable; (2) nurses would be able to modify practices in unpredictable situations and in new situations; (3) valuable practices in nursing will be preserved if the practices are grounded in theory; (4) nurses who verbalize an antitheoretical bias by saying "they know theory but can't practice" would discover that theories are implicit in their practice, if they can be identified, tested, and brought to a conscious level of awareness and utilized by professional nurses. Herein lies the difference between professional and technical nursing.

Theories are abstractions that imperfectly represent reality and are subject to constant testing and validation. Scientific theory is developed by: (1) logical inductive generalizing from empirical facts that identify tested relationships among phenomena, and (2) theoretical "armchair" speculation from which hypotheses are formulated and tested through research. Knowledge is increasing with remarkable rapidity. Man's mind is not exactly like a computer which can store innumerable facts about concrete items. Man's mind has the ability to generalize, to discriminate and identify relationships.

If nurses expect to continue to be recognized as professionals and maintain a respected position in the academic community, and above all provide nursing care for the public, three problems require some kind of resolution. The problems are: (1) antitheoretical bias in nursing; (2) dearth of concept identification and development for nursing that serve as building blocks for theory development; (3) the unknown domain of nursing theory which, in the writer's opinion, will emerge as a science of human behavior.

Criteria for Evaluating a Theory

The following criteria were selected from the writings of several theorists in the philosophy of science and in behavioral sciences.

1. The language of the theory—the terms used—the verbal symbols. Concept formation deals with words and their meaning. What are the terms of the theory?

2. Are the terms defined for operational purposes, that is, for formulating hypotheses, for the readers to understand the meaning.

3. Does the content of the theory approach the characteristics of science, that is, certainty, structure, generalizations?

4. Are the terms universal, that is, applicable to all members of a class, or are they specific and thus limited in time and place?

5. What research findings have been reported to verify the concepts or to test the theoretical basis presented?

6. Does the theoretical formulation contain the following components:
   a. A set of postulates (assumptions)
   b. Basic terms (concepts) defined
   c. A model or abstract representation for the postulates
   d. Rules of correspondence

7. Is the theory generalizable; that is, is it abstract?

8. What are the specific events it explains?

9. Is it limited by time and place?

10. Is it useful in adding to one's understanding of the world and of the field of nursing?

An adequate theory will be generalizable, hence abstract; the broader the range of specific events it explains, the more powerful the theory; it cannot be limited by time or place. The ultimate criterion of a scientific theory is its utility in adding to one's understanding of man and his environment and the complexity of nursing situations in which nurses practice today.

A conceptual frame of reference provides categories or a set of interrelated concepts that specifies variables and constants, whose specific values are determined empirically. The definitions of the terms must be logically consistent with one another, yet represent independent constituents of sensory experience.

A General Framework for Nursing

A personal concern about the changes influencing nursing, a conscious awareness of the knowledge explosion, and a hunch that some of the essential components of nursing have persisted over time, have prompted the exploration of several questions.

1. What are some of the social and educational changes in the United States that have influenced changes in nursing?
2. What basic elements are continuous throughout these changes in nursing?
3. What is the scope of the practice of nursing, and in what kind of settings do nurses perform their functions?
4. Are the current goals of nursing similar to those of the past half century?
5. What are the dimensions of practice that have given the field of nursing a unifying focus over time?

These questions established a framework for thinking about nursing today, for reading about nursing in society, for discussing ideas with nurses and other individuals. Several thoughts were consistently expressed: that nursing is complex because of the human variables in nursing situations; that nurses play many roles in social institutions of varying sizes, organization, and with a variety of persons; and that the past and the present influence the responsibilities and decisions made by nurses. These ideas prompted the exploration of the relatively new field of systems analysis, general systems theory, and another series of questions.

1. What kind of decisions are nurses required to make in the course of their roles and responsibilities?
2. What kind of information is essential for them to make decisions?
3. What are the alternatives in nursing situations?
4. What alternative courses of action do nurses have in making critical decisions about another individual's care, recovery, and health?

5. What skills do nurses now perform and what knowledge is essential for nurses to make decisions about alternatives?

In moving toward the identification of a general theory for nursing, concepts that consistently appeared in nursing literature, in research findings, in speeches by nurses and were observable in

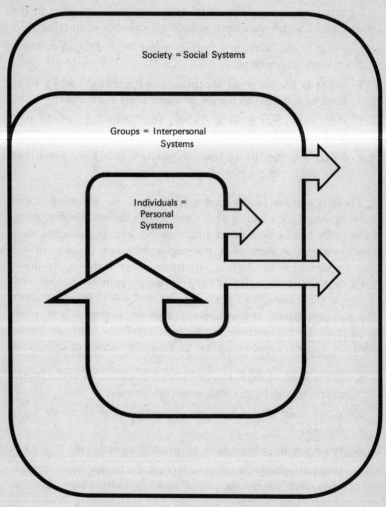

Society = Social Systems

Groups = Interpersonal Systems

Individuals = Personal Systems

FIGURE 2-1.   Dynamic interacting systems.

the world of nursing practice were identified and synthesized into a conceptual framework.

Nurses work with individuals and with groups. They perform their functions within social systems. Three distinct levels of operation exist: (1) the individual, (2) the group, and (3) society. These levels of analysis are conceived to be dynamic interacting systems as shown in Figure 2-1. The unit of analysis in this configuration is human behavior.

Nurses use words, gestures, and actions to communicate information and to establish relationships with many individuals in nursing situations. Analysis of word symbols and of natural situations provides a means for identifying underlying concepts that have meaning for nurses, for the recipient of nursing care, and assist in identifying basic elements in nursing practice. It is imperative that nurses be aware of the potential disparity that often exists between the referent (behaviors symbolized in the concept) and the reference (meaning to the individual).

Level of Functions	Systems	Basic Concepts
Society	Social systems	Social organization role, status
Groups	Interpersonal systems	Interpersonal relations communication
Individuals	Personal systems	Perception information, energy

FIGURE 2-2. Basic concepts of functions of systems.

Four universal ideas in Figure 2-2, *social systems, health, perception,* and *interpersonal relations,* have been selected for exploration because they apply to all human beings and represent to the author sources of the conceptual base of the dimensions of nursing; that is, the physical, emotional, social, and intellectual state and capacity of individuals and groups encountered by nurses. Each of these ideas represents dynamic interacting processes, and are discussed in subsequent chapters. Concepts underlying these ideas are implict in current practice of some professionals. Each of the ideas encompasses a wide range of phenomena whereby isolated and fragmented facts can be subsumed under these generalizations.

The selection of the above word symbols was based on a belief about nursing: nurses, in the performance of their roles and responsibilities, assist individuals and groups in society to attain, maintain, and restore health. In the process of functioning in social institutions, nurses assist individuals to meet their basic needs at some point in time in the life cycle when they cannot do this for themselves. An understanding of basic human needs in the physical, social, emotional, and intellectual realm of the life process from conception to old age, within the context of social systems of the culture in which nurses live and work, is essential and basic content for learning the practice of nursing.

Definition of the Concepts

Man functions in *social systems* through *interpersonal relationships* in terms of his *perceptions* which influence his life and his *health*. The framework is social systems; the methods are interpersonal relationships; the determinants are perception and health. Figure 2-3 depicts these ideas.

Social Systems

Groups of individuals join together in a network or system of social relationships to achieve common goals developed about a system of values with an organized set of practices and the methods to regulate practices and administer the rules. The members of the groups interact according to standards or norms based on a set of roles and status. Certain structural and functional characteristics are found in all social systems such as values, behavior patterns, prescribed roles, status, authority and age gradation.

Perception

Perception is each individual's representation or image of reality; an awareness of objects, persons, and events. Allport and Bruner note that perceptual theory and learning theory are two different ways of looking at the same facts.

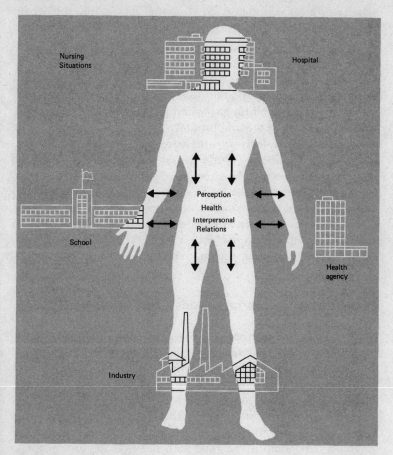

FIGURE 2-3. Frame of reference. Man—Health—Perception—Interpersonal Relations—Social Systems.

Interpersonal Relations

The interaction of two or more individuals in the existential moments in time for some purpose or goal is called an interpersonal relation. In reference to nurse-client relations, the relationship is viewed as a functional closeness between two individuals, usually strangers, who bring to the nursing situation their individual expectations, goals, needs, and values. Implicit in this relationship is a concept of action. Action deals with control over and responsibility for events that transpire in the environment.

Health

Health is a dynamic state in the life cycle of an organism which implies continuous adaptation to stresses in the internal and external environment through optimum use of one's resources to achieve maximum potential for daily living. Health relates to the way an individual deals with the stresses of growth and development while functioning within the cultural pattern in which he was born and to which he attempts to conform.

The four terms selected and defined represent fundamental concepts in the frame of reference presented here for nursing. These concepts are basic in any field of practice that involves an interaction of persons to achieve a goal. What relationship does this framework have for nursing specifically?

Definitions of Terms in Nursing

Man, the human organism, is the central focus for the framework. Environment, internal and external, are essential factors in the human organism's adaptation to life and health. Nurses in the course of their professional responsibilities influence the environment and exert some control over it.

Nursing situation is conceived to be the immediate environment, spatial and temporal reality, in which nurse and client establish a relationship to cope with health states and adapt to changes in activities of daily living if the situation demands adjustment.

Nursing act is like all other human acts, a sequence of behaviors of interacting persons that occur in the following three phases:

1. Recognition of presenting conditions
2. Operations or activities related to the conditions or situations
3. Motivation to exert some control over the events to achieve goals

Nursing process is a series of acts which connote action, reaction, interaction. Transaction follows when a reciprocal relationship is established by nurse and client in which both actively participate in determining goals to be achieved in specific nursing situations.

Nursing is a process of action, reaction, interaction, and transaction, whereby nurses assist individuals of any age and socioeconomic group to meet their basic needs in performing activities of daily living and to cope with health and illness at some particular point in the life cycle.

Need is a state of energy exchange within and external to the human organism that leads to behavioral responses to situations, events, and persons. Behavioral responses can be observed and inferences made about a need of an individual.

The framework identifies three systems rather than component parts of systems. *Personal systems* describe *individuals* in which a fundamental concept is *perception*. *Interpersonal systems* describe *groups* in which a basic concept is *interpersonal relations*. *Social systems* describe *society* in which individuals form groups to carry on activities of daily living to maintain life and *health*.

Hospitals are one of the social systems established to care for individuals who require assistance to cope with their health state or change in health state due to a crisis such as illness. The individual needing this kind of assistance enters the health care system such as a hospital and thus comes to a nursing situation.

A diagram of the nursing process in Figure 2-4 shows a dyadic relationship between nurse and health client in which both individuals are perceiving the other simultaneously, making judgments and formulating in this mental process some kind of action. Direct observations can be made of the reaction of these two individuals from which one infers the mental action. This is a continuous dynamic process rather than separate incidents in which the verbal and nonverbal responses of one person influence the perception and the responses of the other person and vice versa. These are simultaneous acts that are inferred from direct observation of presenting behavior of individuals in any situation. The process shown here holds true in any interaction in which two or more persons meet. Where does all of this information lead us? It indicates the interrelationship between individuals and per-

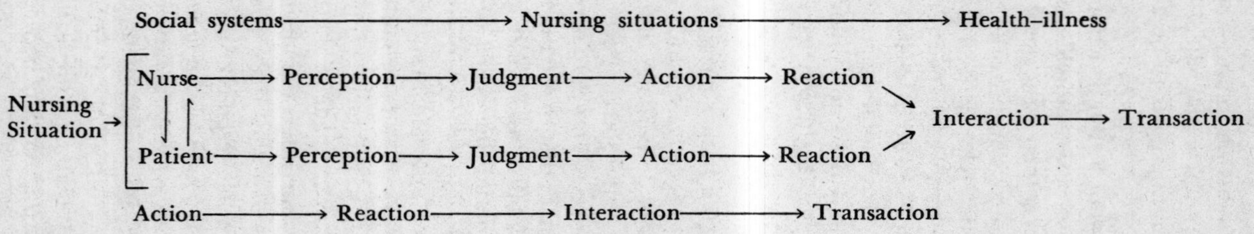

FIGURE 2–4. The human process—A method for studying nursing process.

26

sonal systems, groups and interpersonal systems, society and social systems. Ways to study systems rather than components or isolated parts of systems are appropriate methodology for nursing. Today, nurses are asked to solve problems in complex interacting systems, such as staff problems in nursing service or patient problems involving many individuals and objects in the environment, and nurses are expected to predict what will happen and make a decision for action and thus prevent problems from occurring and plan to adapt to emergencies of life. What theories, models, and methods can be developed and utilized in making decisions for action in complex interacting systems, namely health care systems? The conceptual framework presented in this volume is one approach to the current problem. In any empirical science, the task is to observe, describe, and classify events in a systematic way.

Summary

In any discussion of the nature of nursing, the central theme revolves around man and his environment. Implicit in this theme is a concept of energy. A need for formulating conceptual frames of reference for nursing was discussed. In looking for a common language that allows the representation of multiple facts in nursing, a few basic concepts, which occur again and again in nursing literature, in reported nursing research, in conferences, and in observations in the real world of nursing, can provide a way of organizing ideas for cognitive economy.

The use of the terms concept and theory have been explained and selected criteria for evaluating theories were identified. An overview of a frame of reference for nursing practice relative to conceiving the individual, the group, and society as dynamic interacting systems identified four major concepts. The four terms, social systems, perception, interpersonal relations, and health, are abstract, explain a broad range of specific events, are not limited by time or place, and are interrelated. The relationship of these terms to nursing are developed in subsequent chapters; however, the definitions of the terms in nursing were given.

The conceptual frame of reference can serve as a means of communication as nurses consider simultaneously man and his world in health and illness. Moreover, this framework can be used by teachers in higher education to develop a first course or sequence of courses in nursing as a theoretical foundation for professional nursing. Furthermore, a conceptual framework is useful in planning for patient care and in studying professional nursing practice. As more nurses conduct research in nursing, the findings will sharpen and clarify differences between nursing and other practice disciplines.

Selected Readings

Ausubel, David P., *The Psychology of Meaningful Verbal Learning*, Grune and Stratton, New York, 1963.

Bailey, D. E., "Clinical Inference in Nursing—Analysis of Nursing Action Patterns," *Nursing Research*, Spring 1967, pp. 154-160.

Batey, Marjorie V. (ed.), *Communicating Nursing Research*, Western Interstate Commission for Higher Education, Boulder, Colo., 1968.

Brodt, Dagmar, "A Synergistic Theory of Nursing," *American Journal of Nursing*, August 1969, p. 1674.

Buber, Martin, *I and Thou*, Charles Scribner's Sons, New York, 1958.

Davis, N. S., "Variations in Patient's Compliance with Doctors Advice—An Empirical Analysis of Patterns of Communication," *American Journal of Public Health*, February 1968, pp. 274-288.

DeChardin, Pierre Teilhard, *The Future of Man*, Harper & Row, New York, 1964.

Dickoff, James, and James, Patricia, The Fourth Inter-university Faculty Work Conference, *Physical-Biological Bases for Nursing Care*, New England Council on Higher Education for Nursing, Durham, N. H., 1967, pp. 11-30.

Dickoff, James; James, Patricia; and Wiedenbach, Ernestine, "Theory in a Practice Discipline: Part I. Practice Oriented Theory," *Nursing Research*, September-October 1968, pp. 415-435.

————— "Theory in a Practice Discipline: Part II. Practice Oriented Research," *Nursing Research*, November-December 1968, pp. 545-554.

Dodge, Joan, "Factors Related to Patient's Perceptions of their Cognitive Needs," *Nursing Research*, November-December 1969, pp. 502-513.

Dubos, Rene, *The Torch of Life*, Pocket Books, New York, First Printing, 1963.

Feigl, Herman, and Brodbeck, M. (eds.), *Readings in the Philosophy of Science*, Appleton Century Crofts, New York, 1953.

Goffman, Erving, *The Presentation of Self in Everyday Life*, Doubleday Anchor Books, Garden City, N. Y. 1959.

Grazia, Alfred de, and Sohn, David A. (eds.), *Revolution in Teaching: New Theory, Technology, and Curricula*, Bantam Books, New York, 1964.

Kilpatrick, F. P. (ed.), *Human Behavior from the Transactional Point of View*, Institute for Associated Research, Hanover, N. H., 1952.

Nurnberger, John I., M.D., et al., *An Introduction to the Science of Human Behavior*, Appleton Century Crofts, New York, 1963.

Priestley, J. B., *Man and Time*, Dell Publishing Co. New York, 1964.

Riley, Mathilda White, "An Inventory to Research Findings," Volume I. "Implications for the Professions," Volume II. *Aging and Society*, Russell Sage Foundation, New York, 1968.

Smoyak, Shirley A. "Toward Understanding Nursing Situations: A Transaction Paradigm," *Nursing Research*, September-October 1969, pp. 405-411.

Triplett, June L., "Characteristics and Perceptions of Low-Income Women and Use of Preventive Health Services," *Nursing Research*, March-April 1970, pp. 140-146.

Wolfgang, A., "Effects of Social Cues and Task Complexity in Concept Identification," *Journal of Educational Psychology*, February 1967, pp. 36-40.

Zderad, Loretta T., and Belcher, Helen C., *Developing Behavioral Concepts in Nursing*, Southern Regional Education Board, Atlanta, Ga., 1968.

Chapter 3

Utilization of a Conceptual Framework for Nursing

A profession is recognized by society when it provides a social service to meet a social need. Whitehead[1] distinguished between crafts of the ancient world and professions of the modern world. He explained that a craft is "an avocation based upon customary activities and modified by the trial and error of individual practice." A profession, in contrast, is "an avocation whose activities are subject to theoretical analysis, and are modified by theoretical conclusions derived from that analysis."

Identification and initial development of a set of concepts that are observable in nursing situations and are interrelated have been proposed as a conceptual frame of reference for nursing. These ideas are derived from reported research, from nursing literature, from discussions with teachers and practitioners, and from knowledge and resources currently available to nurses. The framework proposed in this book identifies fundamental dimensions of the profession. The next phase, which is not a part of this volume, would be to subject the ideas to theoretical analysis.

[1] A. N. Whitehead, *Adventures of Ideas*, Pelican Books, Great Britain, 1948, pp. 73-74.

The common procedure for individuals who choose to enter a profession is to pursue a formal education program to learn the theory and practice of the profession. The existence of educational programs designed to prepare professional nurse practitioners implies that teachers guide learners in attaining an organized body of knowledge that is useful in the performance of professional activities. The triad of research, teaching, and practice are interrelated elements in a profession.

In the past twenty-five years, research has caused an accumulation of knowledge in natural and behavioral sciences that is unsurpassed in the history of man. Advancement in human society has brought us to an age of increased technology and mass communication, and an explosion of knowledge that has exerted a profound influence on world health and nursing. Research is no longer unique to one facet of society; it permeates the lives of men and will continue to bring change in the world. But what relationship does this have to the science of nursing? It is precisely this: one of the major problems facing nursing is the lack of a systematized body of knowledge from research.

Research in Nursing—Potential Use of a Framework

One criterion of a profession is the continuous discovery of knowledge to advance its practice. Research is one of the means by which nursing meets this criterion. A nucleus of scientists is essential for conducting research in nursing. Until recently, few nurses were prepared to conduct scientific investigations.

Nurses have participated in the research of physicians, natural and social scientists. As more nurses have become prepared to conduct research in nursing in patient care, methodology adapted to the field of practice and the character of nursing research have shown a change in focus. Many studies that have implications for nursing care are being reported in professional literature today.

Simmons and Henderson[2] indicate in a general way some of the reasons for the slow progress in nursing research.

Circumstances have been identified that accounted for nearly complete

---

[2] Leo W. Simmons, and Virginia Henderson, *Nursing Research A Survey and Assessment*, Appleton-Century-Crofts, New York, 1964, pp. 5-6.

absence of nursing research for nearly four decades after the brilliant start of modern nursing. An understanding of the lack of such research in the nineteenth century, the sporadic attempts in the first decades of the twentieth century, and the more recent, almost forced growth in the past three decades, depends upon knowledge of the past attitudes held toward nurses, the obstacles they encountered, and their long and heroic struggle to achieve educational opportunities that make research possible.. Even a sketchy social history of the development of nursing education helps explain the difference between the development of research in nursing and its development in allied fields.

One of the great challenges in advancing nursing as a scientific field of study is the continued search for theories for nursing through concept identification, development, and research. If nurses are to help individuals attain health, one of the areas of knowledge important to safe practice is that of normal physiology. Studies to measure physiologic parameters related to patient states have implications for nursing practice. Lewis and Gunn[3] report a study using a laboratory model in which they evaluated a procedure performed by nurses. The procedure was the administration of oxygen by inserting a catheter into a tracheostomy tube. Their purpose was to determine physiologic effects of this procedure on patients. The findings of the laboratory study indicated that "an oxygen catheter placed within a tracheostomy tube acts as an obstruction to simulated expiratory air flow." This type of study brings to the conscious awareness of practitioners and teachers that the methods they use to perform this procedure may indeed cause stress in patients. These findings offer some direction for systematic observations of patients who are receiving oxygen via a catheter inserted into the tracheostomy tube. This is just one kind of specific activity performed by nurses relative to physiology. Similar research is described, for example, in some of the published reports of research conducted at Walter Reed Army Institute of Research, Department of Nursing.[4, 5, 6]

3 Betty J. Lewis, and Ira P. Gunn, "Tracheostomy, Oxygen Administration and Expiratory Air Flow Resistance," *Nursing Research,* Fall 1964, pp. 301-308.

4 M. K. Ginsberg, "A Study of Oral Hygiene Nursing Care," *American Journal of Nursing,* October 1961, pp. 67-69.

5 Glennadee, A. Nichols et al., "Oral, Axillary, and Rectal Temperature Determinations and Relationships," *Nursing Research,* Fall 1966, pp. 307-310.

6 Ira P. Gunn, Elenore F. Sullivan, and Beverly Glor, "Blood Pressure

One of the purposes of theoretical formulations is to organize sets of elements related to the field of study that are useful in learning the practice of a profession. Nursing, like medicine, teaching, and social work, has been described as a helping profession. Implicit in this idea is the fact that the professionals use knowledge for decision making for action. A profession that does not continue to discover, disseminate, and utilize knowledge declines and ceases to exist.

If scientists gather facts, explain facts, and provide for some prediction about man and the universe, and if art is the application of knowledge, then nursing care can be viewed as a judicious blending of the sensitivity of the artist with the cold facts of the scientist to meet some of the health needs of individuals now and in the future.

The conceptual frame of reference presented in this book can be used by researchers to identify variables that have some influence on effectiveness of care provided by nurses. One example is shown in Figure 3-1,[7] which suggests types of variables that could generate hypotheses to be tested in nursing situations. The next step in this analysis is to gather descriptive data in concrete situations that might provide a set of functionally related behaviors directed toward one or more functionally related sets of goals. The frequency with which different types of individuals exhibit behaviors in any set of situations that are oriented toward achieving a goal, must be identified and measured.

Type I variables in Figure 3-1 may serve as potential sources for predicting nurse behavior. For example, differences in education and experience can be hypothesized to account partially for differences in nurse effectiveness. The educational preparation of beginning "registered nurse" practitioners is a variable in patient care. It is assumed that knowledge, communication, and interpersonal skills vary in direct proportion to the training of the graduates of the three types of programs that prepare for "registered professional nurse" functions.

Measurement as a Quantitative Research Criterion," *Nursing Research,* Winter 1966, pp. 4-11.

7 Imogene King, "A Conceptual Frame of Reference for Nursing," *Nursing Research,* January-February 1968, p. 28.

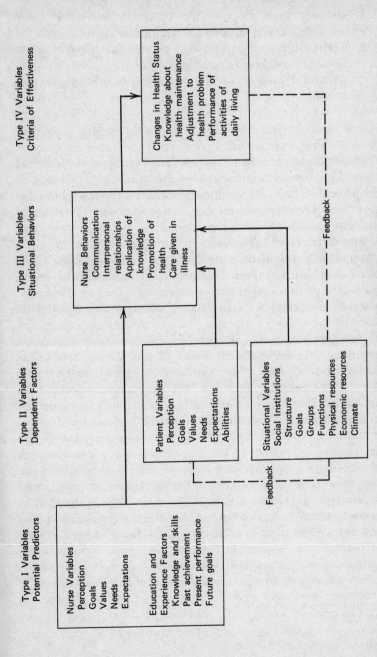

FIGURE 3-1. Types of variables in nursing situations.

Type I Variables
Potential Predictors

Nurse Variables
Perception
Goals
Values
Needs
Expectations

Education and
Experience Factors
Knowledge and skills
Past achievement
Present performance
Future goals

Type II Variables
Dependent Factors

Patient Variables
Perception
Goals
Values
Needs
Expectations
Abilities

Situational Variables
Social Institutions
Structure
Goals
Groups
Functions
Physical resources
Economic resources
Climate

Type III Variables
Situational Behaviors

Nurse Behaviors
Communication
Interpersonal
relationships
Application of
knowledge
Promotion of
health
Care given in
illness

Type IV Variables
Criteria of Effectiveness

Changes in Health Status
Knowledge about
health maintenance
Adjustment to
health problem
Performance of
activities of
daily living

Feedback

Feedback

1. Undergraduate program in a college or university with a major in nursing leads to a baccalaureate degree.
2. Technical program in a junior community college leads to an associate degree in nursing.
3. Technical program in a hospital leads to a diploma in nursing.

One could hypothesize that differences in nursing judgments made by a professional and a technical nurse, reflecting different kinds of education, are directly associated with the difference in knowledge, communication, and interpersonal skills possessed by the professional and the technical nurse. It is further hypothesized that these variations in nurse behavior will occur in different locations in which nursing is practiced.

The variables in Type II have a direct influence on the whole complex of behaviors that enter into the nursing process. Before one can assess the influence of any other variables, the health state to which the individual is responding must be taken into account. An individual's perception of his health state is influenced by his age, sex, class, education, family background, knowledge about health, knowledge about available health services, and previous experiences with illness. A disruption in the biological, psychological, or social process of growth and development causes disequilibrium in a total functioning organism, and necessitates learning new ways of adapting to events and situations in the real world. A social system, such as a hospital, has multiple purposes and goals. If the purposes are not commonly known and accepted by individuals in the social subsystems and if a priority of goals is not clear, conflict will result. The relationship between the patient's needs, the nature of the institution, and the nurse's perception may affect behaviors of nurse and patient. The patient's needs and the nature of the setting influence the values and perceptions of the patient and of the nurse in specific areas of patient care. Changes in behavior vary more often by interactions among nurses and patients and the situation than by differences among situations or differences of individuals alone.

Several hypotheses may be generated about situational behaviors relative to Type III variables. Patient satisfaction increases when nurse performance (action) is congruent with the patient's expectations of this action. Differential perceptions of the nurse and patient directly affect the nurse-patient interactions and the plan of care. If the measure of stress felt by the patient upon hospitalization is related to the sensory deprivation he experiences, then it follows that providing perceptual experiences for the patient will minimize some of the environmental stress of hospitalization. The anticipation of the unknown in the situation often raises the level of tension for the patient. Structured, informative communication of coming events decreases tension in potentially stressful situations. The effectiveness of nursing care is directly related to the number, the kind, and the duration of nurse-patient interactions. If the nurse's actions at the verbal level of communication are congruent with actions at the doing level, patient satisfaction occurs.

The identification of criterion measures to determine the effectiveness of nursing care has been a problem in nursing. Since nurses help individuals and groups cope with levels of health, there is a temporal-spatial relationship involved in determining effectiveness. Health status can be assessed on the basis of goals to be achieved in the limited time spent with individuals and groups, such as measurement of their knowledge about health maintenance, measurement of their adjustment to a health problem, and measurement of their performance of activities of daily living. For example, the goals for a hospitalized patient in the short period of time that the nurse provides assistance are intermediate health goals and can be measured. Studies designed to collect data about the "felt needs" of patients as they perceive them in a nursing situation, and the nurse's observations of apparent "real needs," and the process whereby differences in these perceptions can be fused to achieve health goals would provide clues about some of the basic needs of man in coping with his health status at a particular time. Social interaction between nurse and patient is the independent variable, and individual response is the dependent variable.

If nurses are to assume their role on the health team, it is essential that they have some learning experiences as students that will help them develop attitudes and habits of scientific inquiry.

Concept development in the educational program initiates ways of thinking and means for structuring knowledge for use in practice.

Teaching in Nursing—Potential Use of a Framework

The teacher is an interpreter, communicator, motivator, and a specialist who possesses an ability to help students acquire intellectual, personal, and professional skills. The teacher not only knows the subject matter content, but has some understanding of the nature of learning and of the learner.

A person grows as a total human being and reacts to persons, things, and the environment in an integrated fashion. In the process of learning, a person begins with general ideas and gradually differentiates between the general and the specific. One merely has to observe a child explore his world to make this readily visible. He discovers water, for example, and then begins to differentiate its many uses. As learners are presented with perceptual experiences, they develop concepts. A teacher cannot teach a concept; it is developed by each person relative to his perception. A teacher can, however, discuss his own concepts and those perceived by the individual learners, and thereby arrive at some common attributes or characteristics of knowledge deemed relevant for use by nurses.

Teaching is a process of guiding learners as they build a set of concepts relevant to their selected field of study. **The study of nursing implies more than concepts. It requires another kind of learning—the developing of certain types of skills.** A skill requires neuromuscular coordination and is acquired by regular practice. Psychomotor skills and conceptual activities are quite different kinds of learning, and consequently teachers plan different types of experiences for learners. Conceptual learning is used to make decisions about nursing action, which in turn demands specific abilities such as observation skills, communication skills, interview skills, and technical skills. Decisions for nursing action are made on the basis of one's inferences from perceived data. Often the ways in which teachers guide students through a learning experience are reflected later in the way students guide patients through a learning experience during illness.

In planning a course of instruction, one approach for the teacher to use is to ask three specific questions: (1) *Have the concepts and the skills to be learned by students been identified clearly?* (2) *Have the experiences that offer students opportunities for learning concepts and for practicing skills been selected?* (3) *Have professional values been identified clearly?* The same questions serve a useful purpose when the nurse is planning to teach patients ways to maintain their health, or to adjust to a health problem.

A frame of reference facilitates the development of concepts and learning skills that are considered the foundation for nursing practice. A teacher of nursing recognizes that learners bring to the teaching-learning situation differences in background and experiences. Some similarities exist, too, in that all students have been members of groups; they have assumed many roles in diverse social institutions; they have had some experience with health; and they have been interacting with individuals of different age groups for a minimum of eighteen years. In a college setting they have been introduced to the basic facts of natural and behavioral sciences and the humanities. The first course in nursing complements these learning experiences by helping students relate their knowledge to health and the basic needs of the human being. Part of the course is devoted to a laboratory in which students acquire the basic skills of observation, interviewing, communication with a purpose, and technical skills essential for use in nursing situations. It is in the use of knowledge in specific nursing situations that new relationships are discovered.

Experiences can be planned to provide inputs of stimuli into the students' perceptual milieu that will help them develop concepts and abilities to perform nursing actions that consider the individual and groups. Some of the characteristics related to the individual are age, sex, patterns of growth and development, social class, ethnic background, religion, education, and occupation. Attributes of groups include role, status, authority, leadership, power, structure, functions, communication, and goals. Social systems such as the family, the school, the church, and community organizations have had some influence on thinking and on patterns of behavior of these learners. These factors, and more, have a direct relationship to the four concepts of perception, interpersonal relations, health, and social systems. The influence of perceptual determinants in the learning process is relevant, too, in the teaching process and in the nursing process.

One essential activity of nurses is observation. Teachers select experiences for learners to gain some knowledge of what is to be observed, who is to be observed, and for what purpose. Opportunities are provided for learners to practice the behaviors essential to acquire observation skills and to determine reliability and validity of the observations. Learning experiences may be selected whereby students record their observations of behavior of relatively healthy persons of all age groups. Some of the settings where observations can be made are the school, the well-child clinic, neighborhood health center, health office in industry, and community agencies that promote health.

Moving on from the concept of health, teachers may select experiences whereby students observe and participate in events in which there has been an interference in normal growth and development or a breakdown in some part of the organism. Beginning with knowledge of the basic needs of relatively healthy individuals of various age and socioeconomic groups, they can plan for observation of differences in needs and in behavior of persons who are ill. Illness presents a threat to an individual, and threat is an imposed force that causes defensiveness and constriction in the perceptual field and hinders growth. In order for students to make these types of observations some experiences are planned to identify basic needs of selected patients, and to assess areas in which they require assistance to meet their needs. Some of the settings for these experiences are the hospital, the home, extended care facilities, and outpatient clinics. Time, energy, and planned experiences are essential for students to gain ability in making objective observations, in analyzing information, in making decisions about the plan of care, and in implementing and evaluating it.

Descriptive data collected systematically through direct and indirect observation provide information for hypothesis formulation and testing in nursing situations. This, in turn, contribute to knowledge about human behavior in potentially stressful situations. The learning experiences planned in the educational program, where searching inquiry into the nature of nursing is initiated, will establish the foundation for future learning and practice.

The conceptualization presented in this book may be used by a teacher as a frame of reference for a first course in the nursing major to help students understand health as the life process of growth and development, and interference in the process as a deviation that necessitates adaptation by individuals in the physiologic, the psychologic, or the social realm or in combination. The following outline is an example of one approach whereby the teacher helps students to begin to develop a concept of health.

Concept	*Process*	*Learning Experiences*
Health Operational Definition	*Relating* knowledge from natural and behavioral sciences and humanities to the developmental process of man from conception to aging.	Observe behavior of individuals, groups of different age, sex, class and in diverse social systems using an observation guide for systematic assessment. Test out some of the observation tools suggested by McCain, Beland, Williams, and others.
Specify the Characteristics of Health	*Observing*	Observe ways in which individuals adapt to stress within and outside the human organism. Observe ways in which individuals perform the activities of daily living to fulfill the functions of personal and social life.
	Communicating	Practice structured communication.
	Establishing relationships	Plan for participant and nonparticipant observations along with methods to determine reliability and validity.

Thinking	Identify basic needs of hospitalized individuals, of persons who are chronically ill at home, or the well child and adult. Compare any differences between a relatively healthy functioning person and one who is "ill."
Assessment	
Analysis	
Perceiving and interviewing	Identify the patient's perception of his own needs and his response in meeting them.
	Identify the nurse's perception of patient's needs. Compare the similarities and differences and the ways in which nurses help individuals meet needs.
Measurement instruments to assess needs	Practice the skills essential for performing measurements, e.g., use of observation tool; interview schedule.
Measurement for physiologic parameters such as blood pressure, temperature, etc.	Practice use of these instruments to gain skill in determining accurate measurements of patients' health state or any change in it.
Use concepts to formulate a plan of care based on data obtained	Selected practices to implement a plan of care for individuals, for groups.
Evaluation of plan	Assess whether or not needs have been met or goals achieved. Use available evaluative tools or construct measures related to goals to be achieved.
Reassessment	

The use of measuring instruments, such as the sphygmom nometer and the thermometer, is an essential skill to be learne

The techniques for assisting individuals with personal hygiene, with exercise, and with nutrition are also important in the practice of nursing. These types of skills provide another source of information in the detection of change or interference in the functions and adaptation of the human organism in a nursing situation.

The first course in nursing that introduces students to conceptual learning, and to the tools of observation, and to measurement techniques guides learners in the methods of gathering relevant data. These data and the nurses' knowledge are used to formulate a plan of care for individuals and groups and to implement and evaluate the care given. The art and science of nursing rests with conceptual learning and with the observation, communication, and technical skills necessary to deliver the kind of nursing required in a technological society. The teacher of nursing practice guides the learner as both grow and mature in the process of teaching and learning. In turn, the practitioner guides the health client in learning ways to cope with and to adjust to health problems as both grow and mature in the process of nursing. Change in behavior occurs as changes take place in the perception of self, others, and the environment.

Teachers who guide the intellectual activities of students plan for perceptual experiences whereby concepts can be developed that are relevant for nursing practice. Age is a determinant of roles, status, goals, basic needs, functions, responsibilities, and patterns of growth and development. The length of time a person has lived, the past opportunities he has had for perception, and his physical nature are factors to consider when planning learning experiences for students. These factors are relevant when planning learning experiences for students and for patients. Learners who have had opportunities to explore needs, values, and attitudes will tend as practitioners to provide similar opportunities for patients to achieve the goals of health and perform activities of daily living.

Teachers who create a climate for learning help individuals see things in new ways, explore meanings, feelings, attitudes, and behavior of self and others, and understand relationships between knowledge and its use in nursing practice. Teachers guide learners to maintain a spirit of inquiry that opens their perceptual field to their experiences of the past and present, and prepares them to continue to learn throughout their lifetime, as individuals and as professionals.

Practice of Nursing—Potential Use of a Framework

The primary mission of social-service oriented professions is to deliver a specific kind of service based on knowledge. Professionals from various fields of study may have a similar background of knowledge, but they differ in the way in which they use information in making decisions for action in the performance of their functions.

A case in point is the current demand for nurses with specialized knowledge, ability, and skills to provide nursing care for patients who are admitted to coronary care units, intensive care units, renal dialysis units, and stroke units in hospitals. The complementary and collaborative relationships between nurses and physicians in these units demonstrate that they function from a similar background of knowledge—from a similar frame of reference from which to make split second, and often life-saving decisions. For example, studies of arrhythmias indicate that the crucial role of the nurse (one with specialized knowledge) is not merely one of physical care of the patients, but one of preventing fatal arrhythmias. The use of technology in monitoring patients' physiologic symptoms provides immediate and constant information that is used in detecting signs and symptoms precipitating arrhythmias, and thus nurses' and physicians' action is directed toward prevention. The training of practitioners for this specialized kind of nursing care has been initiated in several centers around the country. The relationship between the discovery of new knowledge from research, the communication and use of the findings in training programs, and the application of this knowledge to practice is obvious in this area of care for patients with coronary conditions.

If this is a single example of specialization in nursing, then what knowledge is essential for general nursing practice which establishes the foundation for a specialized field of practice? An discussion of nursing practice includes assumptions about man a an individual, as a member of groups, and as a part of the society in which he grows, develops, and matures. Nurses learn to record and report their observations in nursing situations in any setting. In addition, teachers must introduce students to methods for establishing the reliability and validity of their observations.

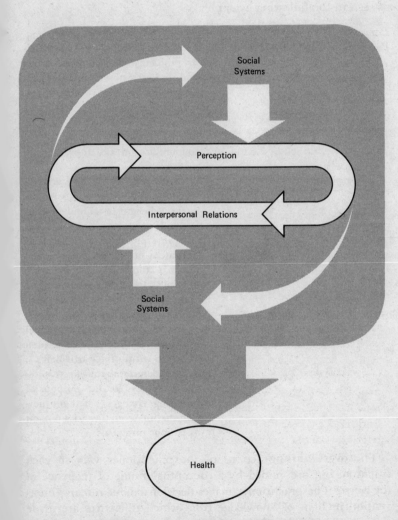

FIGURE 3-2. Interrelationship of the concepts.

The four word symbols offered as a frame of reference for nursing are used by nurses in the performance of their functions. The interrelationship of these terms is shown in Figure 3-2. They may not be aware of this, nor be able to articulate these facts clearly. But the concepts are used as one approach to the identification of problems and to the process of problem solving, as seen in the following example:

Concepts	*Nursing Functions*
Perception	A conscious awareness of the needs or problems inferred from direct and indirect observations of the presenting behavior of individuals. Information about the perceptions of individuals is accumulated by means of verbal and nonverbal communication and the establishment of an . . .
. . . Interpersonal relationship . . .	. . . with individuals. The actions, reactions, and interactions of the nurse and client provide the means for collecting facts. The analysis and interpretation of the facts indicate a priority of basic human needs in the existential moments of time, from which inferences and decisions are made about a course of action related to the . . .
. . . Health . . .	. . . status of the specific individual or group, and carry out the plan of action within the particular . . .
. . . Social system . . .	. . . and determine the effectiveness of the actions for the purpose of initiating changes based on new information and the achievement of patient care goals.

The overt nursing actions of the practitioner vary in each situation, but are guided by a conceptual frame of reference of the nurse. The practitioner makes decisions about nursing intervention in light of knowledge from which inferences are made about perceived data in the situation. A specific example is the use of knowledge in a nursing situation relative to the concept of energy. A nurse who has developed a concept of energy would know about the characteristics of energy, such as its source, the kinds of energy, and conservation and consumption of energy by the organism. A proposition can be stated that oxygen is necessary for life of individual body cells. Oxygen is essential for body cells to convert chemical energy from food to heat energy. When the brain, for example, has been deprived of oxygen for approximately five minutes, it ceases to function normally. If an individual's airway is obstructed and the lungs are deprived of oxygen, death will ensue. These facts are known and have predictive value for a nurse practitioner. Thus, in any nursing situation where oxygen deprivation is observed or where the use of oxygen is essential to comfort or to life, or where the nurse can help the patient conserve energy, the predictive value of this knowledge calls for prescriptive action on the part of the nurse. The perception of the nurse in this type of situation is critical to the safety and comfort of the patient. The nurse's use of knowledge from the natural and behavioral sciences is obvious. Knowledge from other fields of study, and the distinct way the nurse uses it in various nursing situations, necessitates a conceptual frame of reference for the field of nursing that can be articulated by nurses and used as guides to action.

Continued advancement of nursing as a field of study in higher education requires research for the discovery of knowledge and for the questioning of traditional practices. The findings from research that have implications for changing practice must be disseminated by teachers in undergraduate and continuing education programs so that it filters to the operational level of practice where knowledge is utilized.

Identification of fundamental concepts applicable to nursing situations is one way of developing some structure in knowledge, which is essential for nursing practice. Furthermore, concepts can unify nursing through the establishment of a professional language. This, in turn, would facilitate communications and relationships among teachers, researchers, and practitioners as well as interprofessionally, and would move the profession forward on all fronts simultaneously, to chart the destiny of professional nursing.

Summary

This chapter presented a few examples to show the potential use of the conceptual frame of reference for nursing proposed in this book. Several types of variables were selected that indicate some of the complexities in attempting to identify criteria to measure effectiveness of nursing care.

This frame of reference may serve a useful purpose in developing a first course in the nursing major in higher education, upon which subsequent courses may be organized. As students in a professional major are introduced to some fundamental concepts, to a professional language, to skills and to methods for collecting data that are reliable and valid, to analyzing and evaluating information, and to ways of thinking, the basic knowledge and skills essential for practice in a profession may be expanded and improved in subsequent experiences. This book offers one approach for developing concepts with nursing students in higher education.

Selected Readings

Abdellah, Faye, and Levine, Eugene, "Developing a Measure of Patient and Personnel Satisfaction with Nursing Care," *Nursing Research*, February 1957, pp. 100-108.

Bellack, Arno A. (ed.), *Theory and Research in Teaching*, Bureau of Publications, Teachers College, Columbia University, New York, 1963.

Bruner, Jerome, Goodnow, Jacqueline, and Austin, George, *A Study of Thinking*, John Wiley and Sons, New York, 1962.

Bullock, Robert, "Position, Function, and Job Satisfaction of Nurses in the Social System of a Modern Hospital," *Nursing Research*, June 1953.

Carnevali, Doris, and Little, Dolores, "Effects of a Clinical Nursing Research Study on a Hospital," Journal of American Hospital Association, *Hospitals*, September 1, 1965, pp. 70-80.

Dumas, Rhetaugh G., and Leonard, Robert C., "The Effect of Nursing on the Incidence of Postoperative Vomiting," *Nursing Research*, Winter 1963, pp. 12-15.

Ellis, Rosemary, "The Practitioner as Theorist," *American Journal of Nursing*, July 1969, p. 1434.

Hill, Winifred F., *Learning, A Survey of Psychological Interpretations*, Chandler Publishing Co., San Francisco, 1963.

Little, Dolores, "The Nurse-Specialist," *American Journal of Nursing*, March 1967, pp. 552-556.

Mowrer, O. H., *Learning Theory and Behavior*, John Wiley and Sons, New York, 1960.

National League for Nursing, *Nursing Service Without Walls*, Edith Wensley, Dept. of Hospital Nursing, Dept. of Public Health Nursing, National League for Nursing, New York, 1963.

Nursing Research, 1953-1970.

Redman, Barbara, "Nursing Teacher Perceptiveness of Student Attitudes," *Nursing Research,* January-February 1968, p. 59.

Woodruff, Asahel D., *Basic Concepts of Teaching,* Chandler Publishing Co., San Francisco, California, 1961.

Chapter 4

Social Systems—A Dimension of Nursing

The moving forces in nursing are imbedded in the dynamics of society in which the process of change alters the environment. Social forces are in constant motion within social systems, and the interplay of these forces influences social behavior, interaction, perception, and health. Fear, hope, anxiety, loneliness, and pain are a few of the phenomena confronted by nurses in their relationships with individuals in various situations. Nurses are involved, too, on a day-to-day basis with changes in degree of any one or more of these phenomena.

In daily associations with persons from various cultural and socio-economic groups nurses have many opportunities to observe behavioral changes and their effect on themselves and others. Behavior results from learning experiences in the social systems in which individuals grow and develop their abilities to adapt to change. In nurse-patient relationships in health care systems, nurses plan change and participate in the change process through interaction and nursing intervention in selected situations. Some understanding of the health care systems as social systems in which nurses as individuals interact with a variety of health clients and health workers is essential for personal and professional growth. In other words, there are social systems such as, the few examples shown in Figure 4-1 that influence individuals as they

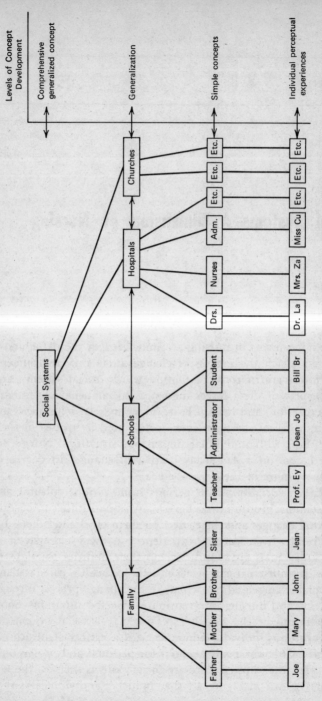

FIGURE 4-1. A way of describing levels of conceptualization from concrete experiences to abstract generalizations.

grow and develop and move into adulthood. There are social systems in which adults function as professionals such as the hospital, public health agencies, industry, school, local, state, and national governments. The settings in which nurses deliver a service vary in size, structure, environment, values, resources, and goals. Nurses encounter a wide range of human experiences in the life cycle of man.

Because of these factors, a concept of social systems as a dimension of nursing is proposed for a conceptual frame of reference for nursing.

Characteristics of Social Systems

Man's biological inheritance and the social systems into which he is born, grows, and develops determine experiences and learning that influence his behavior. Changes in human behavior are exhibited when individuals have acquired new knowledge or formed new insights based on previous knowledge or when there is some interference in the life cycle. Systems provide the framework for social interaction, define social relationship, and establish rules of behavior and modes of action. Beliefs, attitudes, values, and customs are learned within social systems such as the family, the school, and the church. Nurses, as individuals, are like all other human beings in this respect. They function within and are part of many different social groups. The individual social roles comprise the network of social systems.

At birth, the individual makes his debut into his first human group, the family. The family is a social system because it exhibits characteristics such as structure, status, role, and social interaction. Beliefs, customs, and values are transmitted to the children. The family in most instances provides the initial process of socialization for the individual.

The nature of man's institutional life and social groups tends to define types of relationships that he will develop. Many social groups exist in different types of social systems. The pressures to conform to group goals and standards are strong. Reference groups tend to influence the individual's perception, behavior, and judgments.

Eisenstadt[1] analyzes the differences between age groups by relating them to the structural characteristics of the social system and its integrative mechanisms in order to demonstrate continuity in the system. Some of these differences are the life span that the age groups cover, differences between task performance, and types of conformity or deviancy. "Age and differences of age are among the most basic and crucial aspects of human life and determinants of human destiny. . . . It becomes a basis for defining human beings, for the formation of mutual relationships and activities, and for the differential allocation of social roles." The problems of age are universal, whereas the process of aging is biologically and often culturally defined. The adult role is defined very distinctly in most societies. It is a time when individuals become full members of the social system.

Analysis of the dynamics of social systems by Parsons[2] shows the structural bases as the act, the status-role, and the individual actor who participates in a "patterned interactive relationship." The role and status of nurses in health care systems indicate some of the functional characteristics. In addition, the health clients and nurses as individuals have had different life experiences in various types of social systems, and these factors tend to influence behavior, beliefs, and the way in which each individual cognitively structures the world around him.

Woods defines a social institution as the "organized system of practices and social roles developed about a value or series of values, and the machinery evolved to regulate the practices and administer the rules."[3] Within the context of this definition, nurses as individuals learn customs, attitudes, beliefs, and modes of behavior within institutions in the same way as the persons for whom they provide professional services.

Certain structural and functional characteristics are found in all social systems—values, behavior patterns, prescribed roles,

[1] S. N. Eisenstadt, *From Generation to Generation: Age Groups and Social Structure,* The Free Press, New York, 1964, p. 269.

[2] Talcott Parsons, *The Social System,* The Free Press, New York, 1951, pp. 24-25.

[3] Sister Frances Jerome Woods, *Cultural Values in American Ethnic Groups,* Harper and Brothers, New York, 1956, p. 14.

status, authority, and age gradation. Linton[4] has compared the nature of a social system to a geometric figure—"a bit of nothing intricately drawn together." A social system is a configuration of relationships within a culture. Culture is a pattern of living, a way of behaving, thinking, believing, and feeling that is cumulative from one generation to another and that changes in the process of cross-cultural contact. Roles, status, and authority are part of the pattern of living. The settings in which nurses perform their functions exhibit these structural and functional characteristics.

Social class, role, status, and ethnic values appear to be critical variables that enter into social perception and interaction. Some of the sociological studies of the roles and expectations of nurses appear to be related to this idea. Benne's study,[5] for example, of the role of nurses indicates divergence in roles and expectations of individuals. Hadley[6] clearly distinguishes between role and position in a system of interaction. She notes that the essence of the "nurses role," from the standpoint of the interactionist concept, embraces "dependent and independent actions" guided by sentiments of "care, the primary goal of nursing."

Knowledge of the influence of social systems on the behavior of individuals and groups is relevant for nurses. Nurses have multiple opportunities to function in diverse settings and in local, state, and national organizations.

Occupational Opportunities for Nursing—The Settings

Nurses work as practitioners, teachers, consultants, administrators, and researchers in different types of institutions. For example, voluntary and official public health agencies are operated at local, state, and national levels of society. The nursing, medical, and

---

4 Ralph Linton, *The Study of Man,* Appleton Century Co., New York, 1936, pp. 256-262.

5 K. D. Benne and W. G. Bennis, "The Role of the Professional Nurse," *American Journal of Nursing,* February 1959, pp. 196-198; 380-383.

6 Betty Jo Hadley, "The Dynamic Interactionist Concept of Role," *The Journal of Nursing Education,* April 1967, p. 7.

paramedical personnel in these agencies use their time, energy, skills, and financial resources to improve health care and health services for families and communities.

The majority of nurses today are employed by hospitals[7] as staff nurses, head nurses, supervisors, and clinical specialists. Hospitals also employ nursing administrators, teachers, and researchers. The hospitals in the United States are located in rural, urban, and suburban communities, and are commonly called "general community hospitals," or "medical centers," or are specialized institutions.

In these diverse locations, specialized patient care units have been established, such as, intensive care units, coronary care units, cerebrovascular or stroke units, obstetric suites, orthopedic and ophthalmologic units, pediatric units, medical and surgical units, outpatient departments, and psychiatric units. Some hospitals have implemented an organizational structure to provide for progressive patient care, and have acute, intermediate, and self-care units along with extended home-care services. Hospitals are complex social organizations, and heterogeneous groups of personnel are employed to achieve the goals of these institutions. A primary purpose of hospitals is health care service for the sick, but they also provide an environment for teaching and research.

The hospital is described by Wilson[8] as one of the most complex social institutions in civilization. He notes that the social structure involves diverse relationships with predominant roles given to the board of trustees, the administrator, the medical staff, and then to the nurses. Nurses perform the critical service of providing continuity in patient care twenty-four hours a day, three hundred and sixty-five days a year. A predominant role and status in the social structure, however, has not been apparent in the past.

Occupational health nurses have been employed for many years by business and industry to provide health care for adult workers.

[7] American Nurses' Association, *Facts About Nursing*, ANA, New York, 1969, p. 10.

[8] Robert N. Wilson, "The Social Structure of a General Hospital," in *Social Interaction and Patient Care*, edited by James Skipper and Robert Leonard, J. B. Lippincott, Philadelphia, 1965, pp. 233-244.

Emphasis is placed on programs of health promotion and prevention of illness and accidents in the adult working population.

The activities and responsibilities of nurses who work in a physician's office will depend on the physician's area of specialization. A nurse working in a pediatrician's office will deal with children and parents; an internist's office nurse will work with adults; possibly patients of all age groups will be encountered in an ophthalmologist's office; and so on through the medical specialties.

Many public and private elementary and secondary schools in this country employ nurses. Their roles, activities, and responsibilities vary with each school system. Specialized preparation for this very important role of the nurse in child health care is almost nonexistent. Colleges and universities also employ nurses for student health services.

More recently, the expansion of nursing homes has increased the demand for more nurses to direct and supervise care for the aging. Health care programs in several model cities have included the services of a professional nurse as an important member of the health team.

In these various settings where nursing is practiced, health care services are delivered by a variety of medical and paramedical groups, such as physicians, social workers, clinical psychologists, therapists, and technicians. Nurses have performed a managerial function as coordinators of these multiple services, and focus on individual and group needs for care. Each of the professional groups has a role to play in health care, and each professional performs specific activities within the health team relative to his professional goals. Nurses collaborate with the various health professionals on the team to deliver services to the public. They are the persons responsible for establishing reciprocal relationships with members of these diverse groups in the interest of patients and nursing care goals.

Professionals tend to identify with several groups concurrently and to function in different roles by virtue of status and authority. They establish relationships with individuals in specific situations. Qualities considered essential in a therapeutic nurse-patient relationship are mutual trust, respect, and cooperation. Simmons[9] hypothesizes that the degree to which these qualities are "present in a given professional-patient relationship varies inversely with the social distance between participants. Conversely, the greater the social distance the less likely the participants will be to perceive each other in terms of their class status in the larger society." He noted that "extrinsic class considerations tend to overshadow intrinsic therapeutic considerations in the relationship between professionals and patients."[10]

The goals, values, activities, resources, and role expectations of nurses, employers, physicians, and others differ in the various institutional settings and the diverse organizational structures within which nurses function. Nurses are expected to relate with a variety of health professionals. The introduction of new health workers merely compounds the problems facing nurses in social institutions. There is no indication at the present time that the many and varied opportunities for employment will diminish; most probably they will increase. It is important to understand the various settings as well as the different individuals and groups that interact and have been influenced by their experiences in social institutions.

Nurse, Health Client, and Social Systems

Nurses provide a service for a wide range of age and socio-economic groups. The roles and responsibilites of nurses in expanded hospital and home care facilities have increased, and require, in some instances, additional specialized training beyond a basic educational program. The scope of nursing and the different types of settings in which nurses are employed give ample cause for reassessing the knowledge and learning experiences that reasonably can be planned to prepare the future practitioner to operate in such a complex world of work. Moreover, the organizational structure and goals of an institution, and the employer's

9 Ozzie G. Simmons, "Social Status and Public Health, in *Patients, Physicians, and Illness*, edited by E. Gartly Jaco, The Free Press, New York, Chapter 12, pp. 109, 107-112.
10 Ibid.

expectations of registered nurses, may enhance or impinge on the practitioners' ability to give direct patient care. When the values, goals, and sentiments of the nurse are in conflict with the goals and expectations of the institution, the quality of care may be affected adversely.

The individuals who require nursing care range from low to high socioeconomic class, and represent diverse ethnic groups with various religious beliefs and cultural patterns of behavior, and a wide range of age differences, education, and life experiences. Nurses assist individuals who have a need for health teaching and guidance; provide care for those who are critically and/or moderately ill in hospitals and whose immediate needs are essentially physical and psychological; those who are convalescing from illness; those with a chronic illness who require support in learning new ways to adjust to a health problem and be a productive human being; and help others die with dignity. Additional facets of nursing practice are health guidance for the nonhospitalized individual and family, health teaching for the school child, and prevention of illness and accidents in the adult working population.

The professional nurse, interacting with individuals and groups in social institutions, identifies the specific needs of each person in each nursing situation. Individuals hold different values about birth, death, sleep, food, pain, separation from family, body image, status, power, and authority. It is essential for nurses to recognize these differences in attitudes, beliefs, feelings, and customs in order to understand the behavior presented by the health client, and thus to plan for care. Rational behavior in one society is sometimes considered irrational by another group because values are culturally determined. Reported studies have reflected an increased awareness of the relationship between individuals and groups in social institutions.

The concepts of man and society have been related by Knutson[11] into a meaningful whole showing the significance of this relationship to health behavior. He describes the importance of

11 Andie L. Knutson, *The Individual, Society, and Health Behavior*, Russell Sage Foundation, New York, 1965, Chapter 8, pp. 98-116; Chapter 9, pp. 117-131.

recognizing and defining position, status, and role in social institutions. His discussion indicates that communication and learning processes are critical elements in any effort to change an individual's behavior for positive health action. These ideas have relevance for nurses as they plan learning experiences for patients and permit them to practice the behavior essential for learning ways to cope with their health state and for meeting their perceived needs.

A study of social class and mental illness[12] suggests that perception of mental health varies from class to class in the population studied. The data from the limited sample suggest that social and cultural factors can be identified in the majority of treated disorders, but a conclusion could not be reached that these were the essential conditions in the cause of mental disorders.

More people are requiring more health services than ever before in history. Implications for health care are associated with social class differences. How can citizens actively participate in changing their health conditions? How can persons be motivated to see a need for purified water, adequate waste disposal, prenatal care, immunizations, etc., if they have never known these practices?[13] In the last analysis, the health of a community is based on the "ideas, ideals, attitudes, and behavior patterns of the individual and his family, for these determine what he will or will not, can or cannot, expect or accept from those who make his health their professional concern." Class-related differences between the people of a community and the health professionals vary according to perceptions, past experiences, and expectations of individuals and groups. Those factors that enter the perceptual milieu of an individual in a specific situation will determine whether or not he accepts or rejects what is known to be necessary for health.

Some of the studies of roles of nurses, physicians, and others have implied that the roles for which nurses are being educated and the role expectations of employers are divergent. Data from

---

[12] A. Hollingshead and F. C. Redlich, *Social Class and Mental Illness*, John Wiley and Sons, New York, 1958, pp. 357-360.

[13] E. Croft Long (ed.), *Health Objectives for a Developing Nation*, Duke University Press, North Carolina, 1964.

Corwin's study[14] implies that role conflict occurs in the nurse's transition from the educational program to the world of work. The findings of Malone et al.[15] suggest conflict in the role of the nurse in the hospital outpatient department relative to the ideal image versus the real role.

Johnson and Martin[16] view the doctor-nurse-patient relationship as a social system. They contend that the primary role of the nurse is expressive and secondarily instrumental, and that the doctor is the instrumental specialist. They identified instrumental actions as those which help the group move toward a goal, and expressive actions as those related to "maintaining motivational equilibrium" in the individuals composing the group.

Skipper[17] suggests, however, that the nurse's role, as viewed by a limited sample of nurses in one large metropolitan hospital, is a combination of both instrumental and expressive functions. He further notes that insufficient evidence exists to justify emphasizing one function to the exclusion of the other. Dumas and others[18] report results of a study that suggests that the performance of the expressive function (care) and the instrumental function (cure) was essential if the goals for patient care are to be achieved. They report that the performance of the expressive function, whether by the nurse, the doctor, or others, contributes to the instrumental function in assisting individuals through an illness.

Parsons,[19] in contrast, discusses the "sick role" of the patient relative to an institutionalized expectation system: (1) exemption

14 R. G. Corwin and H. J. Taves, "Some Concomitants of Bureaucratic Professional Conceptions of the Nurse Role," *Nursing Research,* 1962, pp. 223-227.

15 Mary Malone, Norman Berkowitz, and Malcolm Klein, "Interpersonal Conflict in the Outpatient Department," *American Journal of Nursing,* March 1962, pp. 108-112.

16 Miriam M. Johnson and Harry W. Martin, "A Sociological Analysis of the Nurse Role," *American Journal of Nursing,* March 1958, pp. 373-377.

17 James K. Skipper, Jr., "The Role of the Hospital Nurse: Is It Instrumental or Expressive?" In *Social Interaction and Patient Care,* edited by Skipper and Leonard, pp. 40-47. J. B. Lippincott, Philadelphia.

18 Ibid., Skipper and Leonard, Dumas et al., pp. 16-29.

19 Talcott Parsons, *The Social System,* The Free Press, New York, 1951, pp. 436-437.

from normal social role responsibilities, (2) state of illness implies a need for help and acceptance of help, (3) illness is undesirable and connotes an obligation to get well, (4) obligated to seek competent help and to cooperate. Findings from studies of the role of nurses and role of patients suggest that many variables operate in social interaction in social institutions.

Some of the legislation passed by Congress in 1965 will continue to influence alterations in health practices, in health services, and in nursing. Research and care centers are being established to apply the most up-to-date scientific findings in the care of persons, and to study factors related to cancer, heart conditions, stroke, and related diseases. Expansion of health facilities has required an increase in the quality and quantity of health workers. To this purpose, the Nurse Training Act of 1964 has been implemented to offer financial assistance to schools of nursing and to individuals interested in becoming nurses. The Manpower Development and Training Act is one means provided for developing programs and for training individuals for positions in the health service areas. The Allied Health Professions Act is another attempt to increase health manpower. The Community Mental Health Center Act, the Comprehensive Health Care Act, the Regional Medical Program Act, and other legislation have given high priority to health programs, to health services, and to the training of health manpower.

Nursing action is concerned with decisions that help individuals move from a state of dependence during an illness to one of independence and interdependence within the social system. Role changes often occur in this process on the part of the nurse and of the patient.

One of the goals of learning to become a nurse practitioner is to gain some understanding of individual and group behavior, and of the differential perceptions and role expectations of self and others. In other words physicians, nurses, and others bring to the situation their own needs, goals, social class values, and expectations as individuals. It is essential for nurses to develop a conscious awareness of the needs, the goals, and the values of patients in order to understand these elements in interactive relationships that influence behavior in health and in illness.

The diversity of social systems in which nurses provide care, and from which their clients come to a nursing situation, require a particular kind of education for leadership in the practice of professional nursing. In the continued search for the scientific foundation for nursing practice, commitment to a singular purpose may well augment the nurses' knowledge and understanding of human behavior. In a profession whose scientific foundation has not yet been firmly established, whose world of work is so diversified, and whose educational system is in transition, the identification of a framework for decision making for nursing action is essential.

Summary

A review of the scope of nursing indicates the complexity of the profession. Nurses are expected to relate with individuals of all age groups, socioeconomic classes, and ethnic orientations in a variety of settings.

Exploration of a concept of social systems as one of the dimensions of nursing has shown that role, status, age, and social class influence an individual and a group's system of values, customs, and behaviors. Nurses employed in complex health care systems often have their functions delegated by their role and status, and this may prevent them from using their knowledge about human behavior and nursing. The nurses' goals for nursing care for individuals may be in conflict with the goals of the health care system. The independent judgments of nurses play a major part in achieving the goal of nursing. A concept of social systems is fundamental in understanding the relationships between individuals, groups, and society, and the influence on the lives and health state of man.

In conclusion, it is the nurses who weave human skills, technical equipment, and administrative structure into a unified approach for delivering nursing and health care within the social systems.

Selected Readings

Argyris, Chris, *Diagnosing Human Relations in Organizations: A Case Study*, Labor and Management Center, Yale University, New Haven, 1956.

Ashby, W. Ross, *An Introduction to Cybernetics*, John Wiley and Sons, New York, 1963.

Bennis, Warren B., *Changing Organizations*, McGraw-Hill Series in Management, New York, 1966.

Bullock, Robert, "Position, Function, and Job Satisfaction of Nurses in the Social System of a Modern Hospital," *Nursing Research*, June 1953, pp. 4-14.

Burling, T. E., Lentz, E., and Wilson, Robert, *The Give and Take in Hospitals*, G. P. Putnam's Sons, New York, 1956.

Churchman, C. West, Ackoff, Russell, and Arnoff, E. Leonard, *Introduction To Operations Research*, John Wiley and Sons, New York, 1957.

Dechert, Charles E. (ed.), *The Social Impact of Cybernetics*, Simon and Schuster, New York, 1966.

Etizioni, Amitai, *Modern Organization*, Prentice-Hall, Englewood Cliffs, N.J., 1964.

Friedson, Eliot (ed.), *The Hospital in Modern Society*, The Free Press, Glencoe, Ill., 1963.

Harrington, Helen Ann, and Theis, Charlotte E., "Institutional Factors Perceived by Baccalaureate Graduates as Influencing Their Performance as Staff Nurses," *Nursing Research*, May-June 1968, pp. 228-235.

Kahn, Robert, et al., *Organizational Stress*, John Wiley and Sons, New York, 1964.

Klein, N. W., Berkowitz, N. H., and Malone, Mary F., "Some Considerations in the Use of Qualitative Judgments as Measures of Organizational Performance," *Sociology and Social Research*, October 1961, pp. 26-35.

Koos, Earl, *The Sociology of the Patient,* 3rd ed., McGraw-Hill, New York, 1959.

Koos, Earl, "Metropolis—What City People Think of Their Medical Services," *American Journal of Public Health,* December 1955, pp. 1551-1558.

Maltz, Maxwell, M.D., *Psychocybernetics,* An Essandess Special Edition, New York, 1967, Copyright 1960 Prentice-Hall Inc., New York.

Menzies, Isabel, "A Case Study in the Functioning of Social Systems as a Defense Against Anxiety," *Human Relations,* February 1964, pp. 54-70.

Merton, Robert, *On Theoretical Sociology,* The Free Press, New York, 1967.

Weiss, James M. A. (ed.), *Nurses, Patients, and Social Systems,* University of Missouri Press, Columbia, Mo., 1968.

Chapter 5

Health—A Goal of Nursing

One of the basic elements in nursing that has remained constant throughout the changes in the profession has been the goal of nursing. In moving toward professionalization, nursing has expanded its frontiers to include not only care of the sick, but also maintenance and restoration of health.

Nurses are individuals and, as members of various groups, have strategic roles to play in the process of human growth and development, and in community planning for the delivery of health services. Individuals in need of health care usually go to one of the agencies where nurses provide care. The social environment in which health care is provided has some effect on the kind and quality of care. For example, an individual with an acute illness is hospitalized for care. In contrast, mothers take their children to health clinics for immunizations to prevent disease.

Society has designed institutions to cope with health and illness. The social legislation passed by Congress in the latter part of the 1960's is evidence of another way in which society is attempting to cope with standards of living, with diseases, chronic and long-term illness, and environmental health. The interrelationship between health, illness, and society is apparent. If nurses in health care institutions continue to define their roles and responsibilities as giving assistance to individuals and groups to attain, maintain, and restore health, then knowledge of biologic, psychologic, socioeconomic, religious, and esthetic parameters of man and his environment is essential for nursing practice.

Health is the second concept suggested for a frame of reference for nursing. Methods and techniques used by nurses to collect information about individuals during episodes of illness have been fairly stable over time. Relevant information has been collected by direct and indirect observations and used to make decisions for nursing action. Selection of alternatives is a function of validity and reliability of observations and information. The more valid and reliable the observations, the more appropriate the decision for action as nurses help individuals to adapt to and cope with alterations in health. Because man is a mortal being, life eventually ceases and death ensues. Although the goal of nursing is health, it is recognized that the roles and responsibilities of nurses include giving assistance to individuals and families during illness, crises, and in death.

A Concept of Health

Health seems to have a distinctive position, a high priority, in the hierarchy of values in society. The establishment of the World Health Organization more than a decade ago and the health legislation passed by the Congress of the United States attest to this fact. **Health is a process of human growth and development that is not always smooth and without conflict.** *Illness may strike at any age and in any socioeconomic group. Identity crises appear at different times in man's life: at the time of puberty, marriage, vocational selection, pregnancy, and aging, to mention a few.* **Health, which encompasses the whole man—physical, emotional, and social—relates to the way in which an individual deals with the stresses of growth and development while functioning within the cultural pattern in which he was born and to which he attempts to conform.**

Illness and health have different meanings for individuals and groups in different cultures. It is known, however, that each human organism has been endowed with particular genes that influence his life process. Although each human being is unique, facts are known about the ways in which the human organism grows, develops, and adapts to change and solves some of life's problems. One of life's problems is the maintenance of a level of health that permits the performance of activities of daily living in order to lead a relatively useful, satisfying, productive, and happy life. This depends on man's external and internal environment working in some type of harmony and balance.

Within the past two decades, especially, disease has been recognized and interpreted in terms of multiple factors rather than in terms limited to a direct agent inciting the disease. This has resulted in an ecologic attitude toward epidemiology, with more attention given to the relationship between the environment and the host. Cultural, industrial, and economic factors have been recognized as significant aspects of health. Thus, along with physical and biological factors, the social milieu is a third component among environmental factors influencing health. In the process of developing a concept of health the ideas of others are helpful in establishing a definition of health, in identifying the characteristics of health, and the relationship of health to the goal of nursing.

Characteristics of Health

Some of the definitions of health proposed by individuals in the health professions have alluded to attributes of health. Tempkin's[1] historical survey of health as a concept has shown that "a feeling of well-being, absence of disease, and ability to fulfill the functions of personal and social life always entered into the notion of health, whether explicitly defined or not."

Dubos[2] notes that human life is a dynamic process and health is an adaptation of man to his total environment, which is ever changing. He moves from a discussion of the abstract idea of health to the reality of life when he states that "complete free-

[1] O. Tempkin, "What is Health? Looking Backward and Ahead," in *Epidemiology of Health,* edited by Iago Galdston, Academy of Medicine, Health Education Council, New York, 1953, p. 21.

[2] Rene Dubos, *Mirage of Health,* Doubleday Anchor Books, Garden City, N.Y., 1961.

dom from disease and from struggle is almost incompatible with the process of living." The title of his book implies that man's birthright is far from complete health and happiness. Morbidity statistics indicate that he is probably correct. A review of some of the research conducted in the health field that might ultimately improve man's state in life, leads one to appreciate that this abstract idea, health, is an aspiration, a goal that individuals continuously attempt to achieve.

When discussing health, Gordon[3] cautions us to remember that we are talking about the total population; as we look around we observe individuals moving on a continuum from wellness to illness and hopefully back to wellness. Gordon proposes that we conceive of a gradient of health, the ideal case of health being juxtaposed to the fatal case of disease at either extremity of the scale. He believes that this shift in movement from well to sick provides some reasons for considering an epidemiology of health.

In the past, a polarity existed between health and illness. Some scientists have been studying multiple factors related to health and disease and data are available that provide clues about these complex and abstract phenomena. The result in a shift in thinking asserts that health is a continuum in the life cycle and illness indicates some form of interference in the cycle.

One study reported that among ninety-five persons over sixty-five years of age, in a low socioeconomic group, the most common perception of health was related to daily activity.[4] Health became important to these individuals only when factors interfered with daily activities and maintenance of independence. This limited investigation offers insights into a few older individuals' feelings about their health. Further study may suggest findings that would be significant in determining health services and preventive care for the older members of the population.

The major ideas found in most definitions of health are included in Romano's definition:

3 John E. Gordon, "Evolution of an Epidemiology of Health III," in *Epidemiology of Health,* edited by Iago Galdston, Health Education Council, New York, 1953.

4 Dorian Apple (ed.), *Sociological Studies of Health and Sickness,* McGraw-Hill, New York, 1960, pp. 37-38.

. . . health and disease are not static entities but are phases of life; dependent at any time on the balance maintained by devices, genically and experientially determined, intent on fulfilling needs and adaptation to and mastering stresses as they may rise from within the organism or from without. Health in a positive sense, consists in the capacity of the organism to maintain a balance in which it may be reasonably free from undue pain, discomfort, disability or limitation of action, including social capacity.[5]

In contrast, Engel defines disease broadly as "failure or disturbance in the growth, development, functions, and adjustments of the organism as a whole or of any of its systems." He notes that his definition permits conceptualization at all levels of organization, the biochemical, cellular, organ, psychological, interpersonal, or social levels of the organism and considers their interrelationships.[6] In this way one does not view disease as something distinct in itself, but rather as related to the individual, his personality, and his environment.

Some individuals have defined illness as a state of disequilibrium in the physical, psychologic, or social components of the total personality. *Illness has been referred to as a deviation from normal; that is, an imbalance in the biological structure of the organism or in the psychological make-up of the organism, or a conflict in the social relationships of the organism.* In this sense, *illness is a characteristic of health.*

Koos[7] raises several questions about illness, its definition and characteristics. When does illness begin? Does illness begin at a point when an individual seeks the advice of a physician? Does illness cease when the physician has treated the individual and tells him he is well again? Is illness easier to define than health?

People perceive illness in different ways in different groups and within different cultures. Jahoda[8] presents some evidence in which

[5] John Romano, M.D., "Basic Orientation and Education of the Medical Student," *Journal of American Medical Association*, 143:409-12, 1950.

[6] George L. Engel, M.D., "A Unified Concept of Health and Disease," *Perspectives in Biology and Medicine*, Summer 1960, Univesrity of Chicago Press, p. 459.

[7] Earl Koos, *The Health of Regionville*, Columbia University Press, New York, 1954.

[8] Marie Jahoda, *Current Concepts of Positive Mental Health*, Joint Commission on Mental Illness and Health, Monograph No. 1, Basic Books, New York, 1958.

specific behaviors are deemed normal or deviant within a particular social and cultural climate. Definitions of illness tend to be understood when viewed within broad sociocultural contexts.

The sick person has been described as one who is admitted to the hospital ward and who is frequently overcome by anxiety because of an actual or symbolic threat to his self-image. Patients commonly fear change in their body image during illness. They fear mutilation and death. Patients cannot anticipate what will happen to them; the doctors and nurses are usually unknown to them, clothes and personal belongings are removed, and the patient is placed in a passive role. These factors, and others, contribute to a loss of personal identity.

Bloom[9] discusses studies that support the fact that although definite signs and symptoms of illness can be described, the meaning of these observations to an individual within a group is variable. Duff and Hollingshead recently reported on a study of the relationship of the care of sick adults from three different "social classes" and the social environment of a hospital. Their study describes the impact of illness on the patient and family; indicates some differences between the quality of care given to lower social class patients and higher social class patients; and highlights the interpersonal conflicts within the hospital setting that affects the sick adversely. They call attention to the fact that sickness is a major issue in society and cannot be dealt with by medical professionals in isolation from society.[10]

Human growth and development can be predicted for each age in terms of characteristic patterns. The internal environment—physiological and psychological processes—work in harmony to enable individuals to adjust to continuous external environmental changes. The developmental processes are manifested anatomically, physiologically, and behaviorally and can be observed, appraised, and in many instances measured. The advances in medical science has enabled physicians to diagnose and treat mental and physical illnesses and to institute measures to prevent illness. Advances in nursing, especially during the 1960's, have emphasized health teaching and guidance as well as care of the

9 Samuel Bloom, *The Doctor and His Patient: A Sociological Interpretation,* Russell Sage Foundation, New York, 1963.

10 Raymond S. Duff, M.D., and August B. Hollingshead, Ph.D., *Sickness and Society,* Harper and Row, New York, 1968, pp. 6-7, 385.

sick. The fact that man has the ability to learn and to adapt t change has influenced the ways in which professionals have begu to view health.

The term health has been used in various metaphorical way Some persons refer to the health of a political party, of a society of a family, or of an individual. Is health an abstract concept Is health a measurable quantity possessed in degrees by all ind viduals? How is health measured when the word is used in s many ways by so many persons? Is health merely a value, an thus perceived differently by each individual, family, and com munity? Many persons have formulated definitions of health others have said that it cannot be defined, but can be described

The World Health Organization says: "Health encompasse the whole man—his total fitness for living; man, in a state o physical, emotional, spiritual, and social well-being, not merel the absence of disease." Although this definition still contain an element of generality, it deals directly with the notion tha health is not simply the absence of disease, a limitation that ha too long dominated the concept of health.

To arrive at some precise definition and measurement of health several questions must be asked: What is well-being? Are ther levels of well-being? Are there gradients of health? Where do w look for health? Can we observe health?

In summary, the common elements of health fall into one o three categories: (1) biologic, (2) psychologic, or (3) social. Gen erally, health is characterized by the ability of an individual t fulfill the functions of personal and social life. The foregoin analysis of various definitions of health and illness identifies som of the common characteristics and the formulation of the writer definition of health: *health is a dynamic state in the life cycle o an organism which implies continuous adaptation to stresses ir the internal and external environment through optimum use o one's resources to achieve maximum potential for daily living.*

Utilizing Woodruff's[11] approach for diagraming levels of con cepts, man and his health is shown in Figure 5-1.

[11] Asahel A. Woodruff, *Basic Concepts for Teaching*, Chandler Publishing Co., San Francisco, 1961, p. 74.

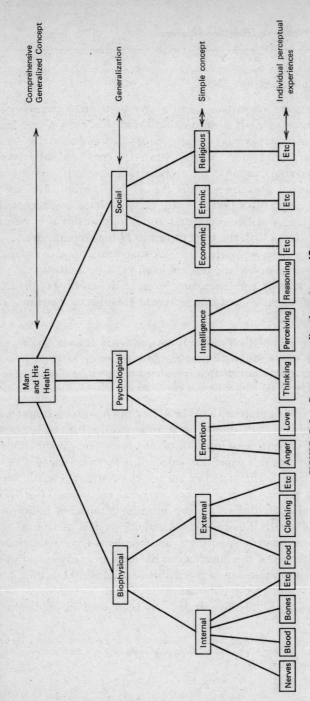

FIGURE 5-1. From generalizations to specifics.

Health Indicators

Most measurements of health have been measurements of ill-ness. One approach to measuring health has been to use health indicators, such as vital statistics, morbidity and mortality figures, and nutritional status. Mortality rate is a crude indicator because it gives no data about social, economic, or emotional consequences of disease; it does not measure the effects of chronic diseases that are not primarily killers. Health services offered and accepted by individuals and environmental conditions within a community are associated with the level of health of that community.

Studies have supported the fact that the level of standards of living are related to the level of health.[12] The fundamental problem of defining and measuring levels of living was explored by a study group sponsored by the World Health Organization. They stated that the

. . . patterns of life throughout the world vary so much that no single standard can be set for all peoples, nor even for the same peoples. But, standards apart, each group is considered to have a level of living which changes in social and economic conditions.[13]

The study group of the World Health Organization noted that "indicators for the direct measurement of health are important; for the present, working indicators have to be sought in deviations from health which are susceptible to measurement."[14]

Available health statistics, such as the National Health Survey provide sources of data on persons and populations. Nutritiona status of individuals and communities is another indicator o levels of health. Environmental conditions such as air and wate pollution, housing conditions, and accidents have a relationshi to health. Since the fluoridation of water in many communitie there is a relationship between this environmental condition an dental health in the population.

The Cornell Medical Index has been used in epidemiologi

12 World Health Organization, *Measurement of Levels of Health*, Technic Report Series #137, Geneva, Switzerland, 1957.

13 Ibid., p. 4.

14 Ibid., p. 23.

studies in America and abroad. This index is a health question-naire that can be self-administered. Abramson[15] discusses its use as an indicator of general health and cites some of the advantages and limitations in epidemiologic studies. The Cornell Index has been shown to have some validity as a measure of emotional disorders. It is considered basically a measure of the way individuals perceive their own health.

Education, employment, recreation activities, and use of health services are factors associated with a level of living. Data from these areas of life in a community may help isolate factors that are associated with health. Health workers need to know how people think, feel, and act as they continue to establish health services and programs that will be useful for and used by the members of a society.

Galdston[16] notes that "the epidemiology of disease rests upon pathology and its associated sciences of bacteriology and toxicology, while the epidemiology of health rests upon normal physiology and its associated sciences of growth, development, and performance."

It is reasonable to assume that the events and situations that prevent disease are not necessarily identical with those factors that promote health. The factors responsible for each of the two conditions, health and disease, are first to be identified and measured. Since health and illness are interpreted as complementary, the common factors that act in both should be isolated. Although nurses plan and give care to individuals at various levels of wellness, they are really concerned with groups of individuals. They are in a position to use epidemiologic methods to isolate those factors that are consistently present in groups of patients and that point to possible causes for events that occur in each patient population. They can use descriptive findings to formulate hypotheses to test in natural situations. If ways exist to define the attributes that are essential to mental, physical, and social func-

---

15 J. H. Abramson, "The Cornell Medical Index as an Epidemiological Tool," *Journal American Public Health*, Vol. 56, No. 2, February 1966, pp. 287-297.

16 Iago Galdston (ed.), *The Epidemiology of Health*, Health Education Council of New York, 1953, p. 3.

tioning, then methods can be used to measure degrees of th
state called health.

A half century ago, most people recognized symptoms of i
nesses because they were infectious and often debilitating. Today
longer life span has introduced concomitant proneness to chron
illness, which may be slow and insidious. In the United State
the younger people have been exposed to methods of health pr
motion (immunization, preschool physical and dental examin
tion, school hearing and sight programs, health teaching) as pa
of the total educational program in most school systems. On
would expect that the younger age group would have differer
perceptions of health than the older persons in society. Their e
periences have been different from those of their parents.

Popular magazines and newspapers impart information abou
health, illness, and new treatments. These sources of informatic
plus television and advertising have contributed to changes i
modern man's concept of health. Today the people of the Unite
States appear to want health information. However, this is ne
sufficient. If health information is to be effective, it must be con
municated in such a way as to motivate each individual to unde
stand it and then to use it. Health education programs will in
crease their effectiveness if they are designed both to give th
public what it wants and to correlate this with what epidemi
logic studies have shown are essential ingredients for health. D
cisions must be based on a plan that combines the goals of th
people with those of the public health officials. How can indivi
uals be motivated to use information to promote health? Th
way in which individuals perceive health will depend on the
past experiences, the environment in which they have lived, an
their concept of health. Beliefs and rituals have a very importar
place in various societies, especially in those that deal with cris
of life, such as birth, death, marriage, and the ceremonial mov
ment from one age group to another. Health professionals, overtl
and covertly, exert some influence on a culture's notion of healtl
especially in teaching individuals ways to adapt to change, an
to maintain and improve their health.

Currently, measurement criteria are limited, as are studies th
identify and measure mental, physical, and social attributes c
health. As methods of measurement continue to be designed

validated, and used, the current arbitrary distinction between health and illness will be more pronounced. Even today, what may be health in one society may be considered illness in another. On the basis of available measurements, a few studies have indicated that there is a relationship between the standard of living and the level of health in each society.

Nursing and Health

Within the past few years, several nurses have suggested that the focus of the subject matter of nursing might be on the components of health relative to individuals, groups, and communities.[17,18] Fifteen years ago a group of nurses, at a World Health Organization meeting, arrived at an agreement about the kind of professional nurse that is needed in all parts of the world: a nurse should be prepared "through general and professional education within her social structure, to share, as a member of a health team, in the care of the sick, the prevention of disease, and promotion of health."[19]

Some of the definitions of nursing of the past thirty years have indicated that health has been an integral part of the goal orientation of nurses, whether or not it has always been explicitly stated or is realistically a part of nursing practice.[20,21,22,23] Nurses, especially during the 1960's, have given more emphasis to the promotion of health and prevention of disease. Nurses have partici-

[17] Grace M. Sarosi, "On the Nature of Nursing and the Phenomenon of Man's Health," *Nursing Science*, August 1965, p. 306.

[18] Catherine Vassalo, "A Concept of Health," *Nursing Science*, August 1965, pp. 236-242.

[19] Ruth Sleeper, "What Kind of Nurse?" *American Journal of Nursing*, July 1952, p. 282.

[20] Effie Taylor, "Of What Is the Nature of Nursing?" *American Journal of Nursing*, May 1934, p. 476.

[21] Martha R. Smith, "A Concept of Nursing," *American Journal of Nursing*, June 1933, p. 565.

[22] American Nurses' Association, "The Biennial," *American Journal of Nursing*, November 1946, pp. 728-746.

[23] "ANA Approves Definition of Nursing Practice," *American Journal of Nursing*, December 1955, p. 1474.

pated more actively in community health planning. They have also begun to consider the total situation, for beyond physiology are the social and psychologic factors associated with health and illness.

Two distinct definitions of nursing are quoted below to reemphasize the goal of nursing. The establishment of unity at this point in time in the nursing profession demands a reorientation to the goal in addition to continuous search for a scientific basis for practice.

The first definition comes from Peplau[24] who presented a concept of nursing in 1952. She noted that "nursing is a significant, therapeutic, interpersonal process."

It functions cooperatively with other human processes that make health possible for individuals in communities. In specific situations in which a professional health team offers health services, nurses participate in the organization of conditions that facilitate natural ongoing tendencies in human organisms. Nursing is an educative instrument, a maturing force, that aims to promote forward movement of personality in the direction of creative, constructive, productive, personal, and community living.

Henderson[25] has formulated the following definitions of nursing:

The unique function of the nurse is to assist the individual, sick or well, in the performance of those activities contributing to health or its recovery (or to peaceful death) that he would perform unaided if he had the necessary strength, will or knowledge. And to do this in such a way as to help him gain independence as rapidly as possible.

She expands the "unique function" of the nurse, saying:

This aspect of her work, this part of her function, she initiates and controls; of this she is master. In addition, she helps the patient to carry out the therapeutic plan as initiated by the physician. She also, as a member of the medical team, helps other members, as they in turn help

24 Hildegard E. Peplau, *Interpersonal Relations in Nursing*, G. P. Putnam and Sons, New York, 1952, p. 16.

25 Virginia Henderson, *Basic Principles of Nursing Care*, International Council of Nurses, London, 1961, p. 3.

her, to plan and carry out the total program whether it be for the improvement of health, or the recovery from illness or support in death.[26]

Basic needs of individuals are usually met within the family structure, but at some point in time and place within any age group these needs reach beyond the competency of the family and must be met by nurses and other members of the health professions. One of the primary responsibilities of nurses is the objective assessment of functional abilities and disabilities of individuals and groups in nursing situations and the planning of purposive, goal directed care.

What difference would it make in patient care if nurses used knowledge about health? In what way would understanding the the use of epidemiologic methods and techniques improve the delivery of nursing service to the public and provide clues for formulating and testing hypotheses in natural situations? What would be the differences in nursing action if nurses were as concerned about the validity and reliability of the patient's pulse, respiration, temperature, and blood pressure as they are when they carefully select instruments and train data collectors for gathering valid and reliable data for research in nursing? Would the quality of nursing care change if nurses systematically assessed factors in the psychological and social environment?

Nurses are in a position to use methods of epidemiology to identify characteristics of groups of patients, various age groups of school children, and others, that will give clues to causes of events that occur in specific populations. In the exploration of a concept of health, several variables stand out: age, sex and socioeconomic status. Basic needs of man and developmental tasks of each age group are an integral part of the concept of health. In an exploration of the nature of nursing, several specific dimensions are relevant: the nurse-patient interaction; an interpersonal process; the nurse's decision about the kind of help clients in a nursing situation require; and assistance given to cope with illness and adaptation to changes in health.

The emphasis in American society on positive health, and the goal-oriented and achievement values in this society delineate two major problems for the health professions: first, to discover

[26] Ibid., p. 3.

methods of helping individuals adapt to changes in health in their life cycle; second, to continuously seek and find new knowledge about human behavior and man's basic needs.

Basic Human Needs

Some of the basic needs of man have been identified as comfort and hygiene, safety, rest, exercise, nutrition, love, sense of security and support, and the need to learn. The three-pronged classification of human needs by Hilgard[27] indicates a relationship between organism and environment in that there are "persistent motivational systems which consider heredity and apperception" and the here and now moments. *A need is a state of energy exchange within and external to the organism which leads to behavioral responses to situations, events, and persons.*

Maslow's[28] often quoted hierarchy of needs indicates that as the organism grows and develops and physiologic needs are satisfied, the next level of need arises and dominates or motivates an individual's behavior. This is not a rigid hierarchy, since there are times when some needs are more prominent and important to some individuals than to others. For instance, for a patient whose physical needs of pain and discomfort are immediate, these would take precedence over his need for self-fulfillment. **Motivation is one of the underlying concepts in a discussion of basic needs.**

A common pattern of health care for Americans who become ill has been hospitalization for diagnosis, treatment, and care during an interference in the life cycle. Several individuals have classified basic needs of hospitalized patients and have developed tools to assess these needs systematically.

At a regional conference for faculty members, Matheney[29] discussed basic human needs theories that suggested implications

27 Ernest Hilgard, *Introduction to Psychology,* Harcourt Brace and World, New York, 1962.

28 Abraham Maslow, *Motivation and Personality,* Harper and Row, New York, 1954.

29 Ruth V. Matheney, "Basic Human Needs Theories and Implications for Nursing Education," New England Council on Higher Education for Nursing, Proceedings of the Second Inter-Unversity Work Conference, 1964, pp. 12-27.

for use in nursing education. All of the theories recognize that man has basic needs and that they influence his behavior. The theories range from distinctly biological or social to a combination of biological, psychological, and social needs.

George and Kuehn[30] studied patterns of patient care and classified human needs that they believed to be common to patients in a hospital. The four categories were: "(1) need for biological and physiological survival, (2) need for safety and security, (3) for love and interdependence, (4) need for self-esteem and esteem for others."

Whiting's report[31] of a study of the nurse-patient relationship offers ideas for further research on basic needs of patients and of nurses. He found that behavior, values, perception, interests, and goals in a hospital setting are influenced and often determined by that setting.

Williams[32] identified seven basic needs (elimination, rest, exercise, social interaction, safety, nutrition, and therapy) and developed a tool for measuring the nursing needs of hospitalized patients. Her approach facilitates direct observations of patients' abilities to perform activities of daily living. It was designed as part of a research project in a hospital nursing unit to measure the nursing needs of patients. Nurses who use this tool can observe and rate the patient's physical ability and behavior response to meet his own needs, and then can formulate a plan of care based on the information. The ratings can give the practitioner data for determining changes in the patient's ability and response to meet his own needs.

Abdellah et al.[33] have presented nurses with a classification of nursing problems. Matheney and others[34] have extended this

[30] Frances L. George and Ruth P. Kuehn, *Patterns of Patient Care,* Macmillan, New York, 1955, p. 10.

[31] J. Frank Whiting, "Patients' Needs, Nurses' Needs, and the Healing Process," *American Journal of Nursing,* 1959, p. 663.

[32] Mary E. Williams, "The Patient Profile," *Nursing Research,* Summer 1960, pp. 122-124.

[33] Faye G. Abdellah, Irene Beland, Alamanda Martin, and Ruth Matheney, *Patient Centered Approaches to Nursing,* Macmillan, New York, 1961.

[34] Ruth Matheney, Breda Nolan, Alice Ehrhart, Gerald Griffin, and Joanne K. Griffin, *Fundamentals of Patient Centered Nursing,* C. V. Mosby, St. Louis, Mo., 1964.

system of classification by using the nursing problems to organize knowledge for teaching and learning the fundamentals of patient centered nursing.

Beland[35] distinguished clearly between the process of observation and the interpretation of observations. She presents nurses with a guide for assessing patient needs and the nursing skills required to meet these needs. McCain[36] adds to the ideas of others about the importance of using an assessment tool, and has developed one that will be useful to nurses seeking to collect relevant information to plan for nursing care. Although each of these guides varies in its presentation, the one element common to all is the necessity for nurses to learn to systematically observe reactions, responses, and events in patient situations as a basis for planning a course of nursing action.

An innovative approach to the study of nursing care of the adult is offered by Smith and Gips.[37] Their frame of reference considers the normal development and change in adulthood as well as the major health problems of the adult. This framework offers flexibility because as major health problems change, so also will the focus of the teaching and practice of nursing change.

Some similarities can be identified in all theories of basic human needs. Needs, overt or covert, are communicated in a wide variety of behaviors. Behavior is learned and thus the need will more than likely be some variation of society's common articulation of this need. Nurses who are attuned to the patterns of behavior in society are able to gain some understanding of individuals and to help them in coping with their basic needs during illness, or other crises, and in maintaining health.

An integral part of an assessment is an exploration of patient's perception of his needs (in situations where this is possible), his attitudes and feelings, his reactions, and his behavioral response to his needs. It is essential for practitioners to have knowledge of normal patterns of growth and development in order to be able to identify deviations. Some of the tools available that were

35 Irene Beland, *Clinical Nursing,* Macmillan, New York, 1965, pp. 20-32.

36 Faye McCain, "Nursing By Assessment—Not by Intuition," *American Journal of Nursing,* April 1965, pp. 82-84.

37 Dorothy Smith and Claudia Gips, *Care of the Adult Patient,* 2nd. ed., J. B. Lippincott, Philadelphia, 1966.

described above can be used as guides for systematic observations in assessing the patient's ability to do things for himself and in evaluating his behavioral response to meet his own needs.

These studies and reports were selected to illustrate that there is very little information about the means individuals use to cope with levels of health. The few methods that are available for assessing basic needs are not used generally by nurses in specific situations to collect data systematically as a basis of planning for nursing action. The findings from some studies provide suggestions from which nurses can continue to gather information about man's needs as they plan for nursing care. Until nurses have some valid and reliable instruments for assessing the basic needs of man, the information gathered will continue to be limited to intuition rather than to a systematic assessment.

Man has three fundamental health needs: (1) usable health information at a time when he needs it and is able to use it, (2) preventive care, and (3) care when ill. An individual's perception of his own health may be different from the physical or psychological symptoms his behavior manifests to others. The nurse is in a position to assess what people know about their health, what they think about their health, how they feel about it, and how they act to maintain it.

The effect of some of the health and education legislation lies in the future. These efforts to improve living standards for some, to help others attain work skills, to beautify recreation facilities for leisure, to control air and water pollution, and to reduce accidents are some of the recent attempts to raise the level of living and health. In addition, the search for an understanding of human behavior may lead to happier and healthier living.

A definition of health remains an arbitrary one until more precise instruments are constructed to measure health states and ways in which persons adapt to changes in health. Further study is also necessary in the complex dimensions of human actions, interactions, reactions, and transactions within the family and other social systems.

A concept of health is an essential dimension in nursing. The dynamics of nursing involve the perception of individuals, and the interpersonal relationships that are established with physicians, patients, families, and other persons.

Summary

The goal of nursing is to help individuals and groups attain, maintain, and restore health. One of the means to achieve the goal is nursing care. In nursing situations where the goal of life and health cannot be achieved, as in a terminal illness, nurses give care and help individuals die with dignity.

The concept of health indicates that illness is an interference in the life cycle and the nurse is a major force in assisting individuals during this period. This chapter dealt with the relationship of health to social systems and presented a definition of health and illness, some of the characteristics of health, and the current status of measurements of levels of health.

Nurses play strategic roles in the process of human growth and development, and in helping individuals cope with episodes of illness in the life cycle. They have an essential role in community planning for the delivery of health services to the public. As professionals, nurses deal with behavior of individuals and groups in potentially stressful situations relative to health and illness and help people meet their basic needs in order to perform activities of daily living. An awareness of the dynamics of nursing is essential if nurses visualize their role as helping individuals cope with stresses related to health states and crises in the life cycle.

Selected Readings

ANA Statement, "Auxiliary Personnel in Nursing Service," *American Journal of Nursing*, July 1962, p. 72.

Annals New York Academy of Sciences, *Epidemiological Analysis of Health Implications of Culture Change: A Conceptual Model*, 1960, pp. 938-949.

Bauer, Raymond A., *Social Indicators*, Massachusetts Institute of Technology Press, Cambridge, Mass., 1966.

Bellak, Leopold, *Psychology of Physical Illness*, Grune and Stratton, New York, 1952.

Cassel, J., and Tyroler, H. A., Epidemiological Studies of Cultural Change in Health Status and Recency of Industrialization, *Arch. Environmental Health*, 1961.

Dingman, Rita, Nursing Action and the Promotion of Health, *ANA Regional Clinical Conferences*, November 1965, American Nurses' Association, New York.

Dunn, Halbert, M.D., "High-Level Wellness for Man and Society," *American Journal of Public Health*, June 1959, pp. 786-792.

Hanson, Robert C., and Beech, Mary J., "Communicating Health Arguments Across Cultures," *Nursing Research*, Fall 1963, pp. 237-241.

Hollingshead, A., and Redlick, F. C., *Social Class and Mental Illness*, John Wiley and Sons, New York, 1958.

Johnson, Carmen Acosta, "Changing Health Attitudes Through Use of Cross-Cultural Materials," *Nursing Research*, Summer 1965, pp. 264-267.

Kasl, S. V., and Cobb, S., "Health Behavior, Illness Behavior, and Sick-role Behavior, I. Health and Illness Behavior," *Archives Environmental Health*, 1966, p. 246.

Lerner, M., and Anderson, O. W., *Health Progress in the U.S. 1900-1960*, University of Chicago Press, Chicago, 1965.

Mechanic, David, "The Concept of Illness Behavior," *Journal of Chronic Disease,* 1962, p. 189.

Miller, James G., "Living Systems: Basic Concepts," *Behavioral Science,* July 1965, pp. 193-237.

Paul, Benjamin D., *Health, Culture and Community,* Russell Sage Foundation, New York, 1955.

Read, Margaret, *Culture, Health and Disease,* Tavistock Publications, J. B. Lippincott, Philadelphia, 1966.

Rogers, Edward, *Human Ecology and Health,* Macmillan, New York, 1960.

Schulman, Sam, "Basic Functional Roles in Nursing: Mother Surrogate and Healer," in *Patients, Physicians, and Illness,* edited by E. Gartly Jaco, The Free Press, Glencoe, Ill., 2nd printing, 1960.

Theis, Charlotte, E., and Harrington, Helen Ann, "Three Factors that Affect Practice: Communication, Assignment, Attitudes," *American Journal of Nursing,* 1968, p. 1478.

Weidenbach, Ernestine, *Clinical Nursing: A Helping Art,* Springer Publishing Co., New York, 1964.

Chapter 6

Dynamics of Nursing

The physical and social environment provides support for individuals to grow and develop as human beings and to move from a state of dependency in childhood to independence and interdependence in adulthood. The boundaries perceived in the life space of individuals give structure to their interpersonal field. In general, people have an awareness of other persons, things, and events in the environment. Perception is a means whereby individuals experience direct contact with the environment. Perception involves the transaction of the human organism with environmental stimuli. An act of perceiving is a function of the human organism in which a transaction occurs between the perceiver and the event, person, or object being perceived.

Events inferred from a person's perceptions give meaning to his experiences and represent an individual's image of his real world. For instance, various types of crises, such as illness, occur in the life cycle of man. When individuals have difficulty in adapting to their environment or when a health problem arises that they cannot resolve, they usually request the assistance of professionals. The recipients of professional services often find themselves in new roles and new environments. The relationships require some adjustment on the part of interacting persons in the immediate situation. The dynamic life process of man involves a constant restructuring of the real world; thus action results from factors in the situation and in the individual at any point in time. Since man and his environment are the central focus for the conceptual framework for nursing, a few basic premises are stated.

Man Is a Reacting Being. Each individual reacts to events, persons, and objects in terms of his own perception, expectations, and needs at a particular moment. Reactions occur in the perceptual milieu of the individuals who are interacting. In other words, we react to each other's perceptions of the situation and to one's expectations of individuals and objects in the environment. Individual reactions to another person or a situation usually occur when experiences in the existential moment are contrary to or exceed expectation or hope. Man as a composite of mind and body reacts as a total organism to his experiences which are viewed as a flow of events in time.

Man Is a Time-Oriented Being. His present has its roots in past experiences, and his awareness of the present influences his prediction of the future. Individuals respond to sensory perception every second as they perceive their needs and immediate goals. Time is an irreversible process in the life cycle, yet the mind of man has the ability to recall past events, to make decisions in the present on the basis of past experiences, and to plan to achieve goals in the future on the basis of the past and present. The transactions, therefore, that occur in human interactions are an exchange of energy and information within the persons involved (intrapersonal) and between the individual and the environment (interpersonal).

Man Is a Social Being. Through language man has found a symbolic way of communicating his thoughts, actions, customs, and beliefs over time. Man can be described in a systematic way by observation of verbal and nonverbal behaviors in different situations; yet he exhibits some common characteristics, such as the ability to perceive, to think, to feel, to choose between alternative courses of action, to set goals and select the means to achieve them, and to make decisions, etc. Man interacts with persons, things, and objects in his environment, and functions within social systems.

An analysis of the dynamics of nursing prompted the selection of perception and interpersonal relations as fundamental ideas in a frame of reference for nursing. "Dynamics" is used in a limited sense to connote adaptive changes occurring in a nurse-client relationship in a nursing situation. "A nursing situation" is conceived to be the immediate environment, spatial and temporal reality, in which nurse and client establish a relationship in order to cope with health problems and adapt to changes in activities of daily living if the situation demands adjustment. A facet of the nurse's role is to help the individual overcome hurdles, to enable him to use his potential ability to function, and to react to the present in order to plan realistically for the future. This implies recognition of the potential ability of individuals, their strengths and weaknesses.

A few factors from selected descriptions of nursing situations indicate that nurses are concerned with environmental factors. Personal factors, for example, include the goals of individuals in the situations, their knowledge and ability to perform acts to achieve goals, and the motivation to exert energy to perform actions. Some of the factors with which nurses deal are the difficulty of the functions to be performed, the opportunities individuals have to work toward goals, and barriers in the immediate situation that may prevent performance and achievement.

Nurses in the performance of their functions influence the actions of the health client. Nurses control environmental factors by removing restrictions on activities of the client, by providing him with information, and by helping him increase his ability to perform actions that will achieve goals. They control environmental factors in some situations by restricting the activities of the client and by withholding information. The client attempts to control his environment in the situation in a similar manner.

The definition of nursing presented in Chapter 2 is restated here because an analysis of some of the words in the definition will be helpful in identifying underlying concepts relative to the dynamics of nursing. *Nursing is a process of action, reaction, interaction, and transaction, whereby nurses assist individuals of any age and socioeconomic group to meet their basic needs in performing activities of daily living and to cope with health and illness at some particular point in the life cycle.* Nurses infer thoughts and feelings from what the client says or does or how he speaks and acts. Interviewing, purposeful communication, and direct observations of behavior are essential skills for nurses to identify patients perceptions. The definition also implies that it is essential for nurses to have knowledge of the learning process, and of the physical, social, and psychological growth and development of all age groups.

Human acts, the behavior of individuals, extend over time and place, and depict various levels of complexity. The perceptions, judgments, actions, and reactions of the nurse and the client will determine the transaction in a particular situation.

The Nursing Act as Process

Nursing acts are goal-directed toward health and can be observed as a process of interaction between nurses and clients in specific situations; they may be influenced by the situation and by interaction with the family, the physician, and other persons and events. The processes involved in nursing situations represent a sequence of behaviors, overt and covert, verbal and nonverbal. When two individuals meet in any situation, some kind of action is involved.

Knowledge of basic elements of action, such as the ability of a person to perform activities, or to see the color in objects, is a part of one's cognitive awareness of facts. Associated with awareness of facts is the individual's attempt to determine the causes of a satisfying or dissatisfying experience. Whether the patient perceives the nurse as really wanting to help him, or as an individual who is doing things for him merely because it is that individual's responsibility to do so, determines whether or not the nurse or the patient make possible a stable environment, and who has the power to control the environment. The factors involved here are the persons and their perceptions of the immediate situation. Purposeful action implies that an individual has control over and is responsible for the events that take place.

Action is a sequence of behaviors of interacting persons which includes (1) recognition of presenting conditions; (2) operations or activities related to the condition or situation; and (3) motivation to exert some control over the events to achieve goals. For example, nurses may recognize overt needs and also become aware of "felt needs" of patients. When the nurse and patient have established mutual interest and understanding of the goals and methods to achieve them, a transaction occurs.

Transactions are considered in Ittleson and Cantril's[1] description of the features of perception:

First, the facts of perception always present themselves through concrete situations. They can be studied only in terms of the transactions in which they can be observed. Second, within such transactions, perceiving is always done by a particular person from his own unique position in space and time and with his own combination of experiences and needs. Perception always enters into the transaction from the unique personal behavioral center of the perceiving individual. Third, within the particular transaction and operating from his own personal behavioral center, each of us, through perceiving, creates himself his own psychological environment by attributing certain aspects of his experience to an environment which he believes exists independent of the experience.

The nursing process is a series of acts which connote action, reaction, interaction. Transaction follows when a reciprocal relationship is established by the nurse and patient in which both participate in determining the goal to be achieved in the specific situation. Ittleson and Cantril describe the term "transaction" as a concrete situation in which the interacting individuals are "actively participating in the events" and this fact of active participation to move toward a goal will affect their identity. The nurse and patient will learn and mature in the process. There are instances when the patient is unable to participate actively in events in the environment. The nurse gives care to the patient and interaction takes place, but there is no transaction unless the above factors exist. In some situations it is not possible for a transaction to occur.

Society has established specific social systems for the purpose of dealing with health and illness. Nurses (and other health professionals) perform their functions in these specific social systems. When a nurse and a patient (or health client) meet in a nursing

---

[1] William H. Ittleson and Hadley Cantril, *Perception: A Transactional Approach,* Doubleday, Garden City, N. Y., 1954, p. 2.

situation, each perceives the other and makes judgments about each other resulting in some kind of action. This action is expressed in verbal and nonverbal behavior resulting in a re- action on the part of nurse and patient.

In the interactive process, as nurse and patient assess goals to be achieved, and mutually define health goals, a transaction occurs. This mutual agreement has an effect on the actions and judgment of the nurse and patient and influences each one's perception. A series of these kind of acts takes place as the nurse and patient interact in a nursing situation. The schematic design that follows shows a sequence of behaviors related to the nursing process.

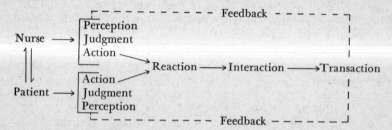

This diagram attempts to show that events in the nursing process influence perceptions of each person even though time is irreversible.

Perception of the nurse leads to judgments and to action by the nurse. Simultaneously, the perception of the patient leads to judgments and then to action by the patient. This a continuous dynamic process rather than separate incidents in which the action of one person influences the perceptions of the other and vice versa. The complex human relationships involved in nursing will be profoundly modified by the nurse's conception of self, man, and his environment. Judgments made by nurses will be influenced by their knowledge of the physical, psychological, and social components of man, by their system of values, and by their selected perceptions in the nursing situation.

The concepts of perception and interpersonal relations are relevant dimensions in any nursing situation because nurses have vital roles to play in the process of human growth and develop- ment in health and in illness. The life cycle of the human organism extends on a continuum that is open and expanding.

When human beings are born, they enter into an already established culture. They grow and develop as individuals within social systems that influence their values and patterns of behavior. Learning and experience influence change in their behavior.

Man's life span is subjected to periods of crises, such as illness, accidents, choice of occupation, and transition from one age group to another. These periods may cause disruptions in one's pattern of living that require adjustments and change. The family, as one of the social systems in a culture, attempts to cope with changes that occur. When the family is unable to maintain its equilibrium, outside individuals and groups are called upon for assistance. A nurse is expected to have the ability to establish an existential relationship with patients to help them cope with their health problem, for example, a physical or mental illness, or another crisis in the life cycle.

Nurses are in a position by virtue of the relationship they establish with individuals and families to study human behavior in a variety of settings and to help individuals learn ways of growing in health and maturity. For nurses to participate in events that help themselves and others move toward the goal of effective health teaching and nursing care, it is essential that they have some understanding of the differential perceptions of health as man interacts with others within various social environments.

During an episode of illness, the nurse makes decisions that promote and implement a plan of care to help individuals maintain and restore health. If health cannot be restored, nurses have an important role to play in the care of the sick and dying patients. They help individuals learn to use the experience of illness as a positive force for personality growth. In the process of responding to the needs of individuals, nurses themselves advance in maturity as they gain greater understanding of human behavior. Perception and interpersonal relations are essential components in the nursing process.

Perception—A Dimension of the Nursing Process

Perception is an awareness of objects, persons, and situations. It is each individual's representation or image of reality.

Although one presupposes that human beings live in the same

world and thus perceive similar things, individuals differ in what they select to enter their perceptual milieu. The perceptual tools, sensory (functioning sense organs) and intellectual (brain processes), vary from person to person. One's perception is related to past experiences, self-concept, socioeconomic groups, biological inheritance, and educational background.

Since one of the functions of a nurse is to help the individual to identify his needs and to establish realistic goals to meet needs, the nurse is responsible for using methods to gain information about an individual's perception of the situation. Through communication, nurses observe and record what the patient says he is feeling or thinking about a particular event. Observations of behavior offer clues to an individual's needs and his perception of the situation. An individual's beliefs influence the meaning he gives to medical treatment, the use of health services, and his reaction to illness, acceptance or rejection of nursing care, and behavior during a particular situation. Measures are available to collect information about patients' and nurses' perceptions. A rating scale, for example, was developed by Palmer[2] to measure the perceptions of adults to impending surgery. The information gathered by using such a scale can help nurses provide perceptual experiences that produce a positive reaction in patients and thus eliminate some of the fear and anxiety of the unknown in a nursing situation.

Heider[3] discusses three sets of conditions to be taken into account in perception: the object, intervening circumstances between the observer and the object, and factors within the organism. He notes that knowledge of these conditions influences one's actions.

Nurses assess the behavior of others on the basis of their own knowledge and perception of the situation. In many instances, nurses demonstrate an intuitive cognition relative to perceptual cues in the situation. For example, a nurse may say that a patient is fearful because "he said this and did thus and so." The raw material consists of the nurse's perception of the actions and

[2] Irene Palmer, "The Development of a Measuring Device," *Nursing Research,* Spring 1965, pp. 100-105.

[3] Fritz Heider, *The Psychology of Interpersonal Relations,* John Wiley and Sons, New York, 1958, pp. 60-70.

reactions of the patient. Generally, the nurse and the patient react to what each one says or does in addition to what they think the other is perceiving. Nurses' and patients' values, attitudes, and beliefs influence their evaluation of a situation. In other words, perception influences one's evaluation of a situation and evaluation influences perception.

In order for nurses to interpret actions and reactions of others, it is essential that they recognize the elements in the perceptual milieu that motivate or hinder achievement of goals. What are the private concerns of health clients, of patients? How do they define the situation? What subjective facts exist for them in this situation? Do we understand the patient's life space, the person, and the psychological environment that exist for him? What are the private concerns of nurses, doctors, and relevant others? How do they define the here and now situation? What are their subjective and objective facts and are they related to the clients? To what extent are their subjective facts in agreement with or in opposition to the subjective facts of the patient they are seeking to understand and to help?

Broad classifications of perceptual determinants discussed by several persons reinforce Kaufmann's ideas.[4] King,[5] for example, presents members of the health professions with a frame of reference in which concepts are selected from the natural and behavioral sciences and supported by some empirical findings. Psychologic factors are categorized as (1) psychologic needs, (2) adaptive and defense mechanisms, and (3) beliefs, attitudes, and values. Examples of physiologic factors are hunger, thirst, and fatigue. Some of the sociocultural factors that determine an individual's perception are the status in the family, and in the world of work and recreation. Status determines role, and this is influenced by variables such as age, sex, education, occupation, income, and social class.

A particular role in a situation usually has concomitant expectations, rights, and duties. For example, the patient's perception

[4] Margaret Kaufmann, *Identification of Theoretical Bases for Nursing Practice,* Unpublished doctroal dissertation, University of California, Los Angeles, 1958.

[5] Stanley H. King, *Perceptions of Illness and Medical Practice,* Russell Sage Foundation, New York, 1962, p. 32.

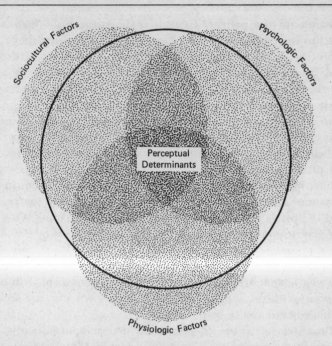

FIGURE 6-1.   Interrelationship of factors determining perception.

of the role of the nurse or the physician and his expectations of them in the performance of the role often influences his behavior. When an individual does not conform to another's expectations of him, conflict may result. This leads to stress and anxiety on the part of each individual. Figure 6-1 shows the interrelatedness of psychologic, sociocultural, and physiologic factors that determine perception.

Psychologic variables tend to influence not only the action and reaction of individuals, but also the interaction between the health professional and the recipient of professional services. When an individual enters a nursing situation, he brings his own needs, background of experiences, words, ideas, beliefs, and prejudices, and these are communicated in a variety of ways through his behavior. Needs can be defined biologically, psychologically, and socially. A need is a state of energy exchange within and external to the organism which leads to behavioral responses to situations, events, and persons. The nurse's perception of basic needs of the patient through observation and purposeful communication often determines the relationship established between the nurse and the patient.

Interpersonal Relations—A Dimension of the Nursing Process

Nursing involves thinking, relating, judging, and acting relative to the health status manifested in the behavior of individuals and groups. Nurses function daily in a laboratory of interpersonal relations. The kind of relationships established with physicians and individuals in allied health professions differ from those initiated with the patient and his family.

In a technological society, where specialization is the rule rather than the exception, health maintenance and delivery of effective health services require both an individual and a team approach. This does not occur in all places and is not possible in some situations. Nevertheless, imperative in the team approach is the establishment and maintenance of a professional relationship that includes open communication among members of the team and a mutual respect for each one's abilities to contribute to the total plan of care. This involves a cooperative and collaborative relationship among members of the health team to achieve goals with and for patients, and to raise the level of health for individuals in the community.

In contrast, a nurse-patient relationship is viewed as a functional closeness between two individuals, usually strangers, who bring to the nursing situation their individual expectations, goals, needs and values. In most instances, the patient comes to a setting in which nurses function. The nurse establishes a relationship with the individual to explore some of the presenting health problems and to give information about the setting and some of the activities to be anticipated in the new environment. Implicit in this relationship is a *concept of action*. Action deals with control over and responsibility for events that transpire in the environment. These relationships provide perceptual experiences for both the nurse and the patient as they develop skills in solving the difficulties that occur relative to the presenting problem. Legal and social status may determine in some instances what persons can or will do. Knowledge, ability, and expectations of the nurse and patient determine actions and reactions in nursing situations.

The interpersonal relations between nurse and patient involve learning experiences whereby two people interact to face an immediate health problem, to share, if possible, in resolving it, and to discover ways to adapt to the situation. In instances of chronic illness, methods are explored for adjusting activities of daily living to cope with the problem; in terminal illness and when death is imminent, nurses help individuals die with dignity.

Each individual brings to the nursing situation his own needs and goals. If the situation permits, a relationship is established whereby the nurse and the patient work together to understand the problem, to learn ways to solve it, and to be able to cope with similar difficulties if they arise in the future. Nurses help patients express their concerns and assist them in using their abilities to recover from illness and to attain and maintain health. They help individuals identify and understand facets of the problem so that energy can be channeled toward positive action. When mutual interest is present in the situation, and when some common understanding is gained of the goals to be achieved, a transaction results.

Peplau's[6] conceptual frame of reference for nursing suggests an interpersonal process as part of a theory of nursing practice. She notes that "clinical nursing science can contribute original insights concerning what happens among human beings who seek help when undergoing stress." She identifies methods for studying nurse-patient relationships and explains some of the basic principles of interpersonal relations in nursing, which also guide one's relations with other professionals and in daily living. Central to Peplau's ideas is the thought that *both the nurse and the patient learn from the relationship* and move toward maturity as a result of it.

Rotter[7] emphasizes the need for knowledge of the psychological

[6] Hildegard E. Peplau, *Interpersonal Relations in Nursing*, G. P. Putnam's Sons, New York, 1952, p. 261.

[7] Julian B. Rotter, *The Role of the Psychological Situation in Determining the Direction of Human Behavior*, Nebraska Symposium on Motivation, University of Nebraska, Lincoln, 1955, pp. 245-268.

situation that would give cues for understanding human behavior. He proposes a social learning theory in which he selects three constructs, behavior potential, expectancy, and reinforcement value.[8]

Allport notes[9] that perceptual theory and learning theory are two different ways of looking at the same facts. Bruner adds emphasis to this idea when he states that "one of the principal characteristics of perceiving is a characteristic of cognition generally."[10] Learning theory is important in any consideration of the nursing process because one's knowledge influences behavior, and this has relevance for actions, reactions, and interactions of nurse and patient.

Human beings, for example, are constantly demonstrating in their behavior many ways in which they attempt to control their environment. When they enter a new setting or when they interact with strangers, their perception of persons and events influences their actions and reactions in the situation. In a nurse-patient relationship, nurses have control over information (the way in which patients encounter information) and, therefore, control the environment. The reverse also operates in that a patient can give or withhold information that may be relevant to his plan of care in an effort to control his environment.

If nurses are to understand behavior and help alleviate stress and anxiety in nursing situations, it is essential that they be aware of the cognitive, affective, and directive aspects involved in the nurse-patient relationship. It is essential, too, that nurses gain some understanding of the various facets of the different types of social systems that impinge upon the patient, the nurse, and others in the environment. Nurses, who structure communication and information, tend to guide individuals to recognize their health needs, to express their feelings about meeting them, and to share in decisions about the means and the goals to be achieved.

Whiting[11] studied needs, values, perceptions, and the nurse-

8 Ibid.

9 Floyd Allport, *Theories of Perception and the Concept of Structure,* John Wiley and Sons, New York, 1955, p. 463.

10 From Beardslee and Wertheimer, *Readings in Perception,* Copyright 1958, D. Van Nostrand Company, Inc., Princeton, New Jersey, p. 687 (per letter from publisher to use quote).

11 J. Frank Whiting, "Q-Sort Technique for Evaluating Perceptions of Interpersonal Relationships," *Nursing Research,* October 1955, p. 71.

patient relationship in a modern hospital. He noted that the "nature of the setting in which the nurse-patient relationship takes place has an influence on the values and perception people hold concerning their own and other's behavior within the setting." The study of behavioral phenomena in natural settings, as reported by Whiting and others, can open up many avenues for nursing research and is essential to evaluate the effectiveness of nursing care.

Howland's[12] hospital system model is another approach used in studying natural situations. His use of cybernetic concepts in the analysis of systems is an attempt to describe ways of integrating information, regulation, and control in the complex social system of the hospital. Who makes the decisions that may enhance or impinge on the plan of care for patients? How, when, and where are these decisions made? Cybernetics deals with function and behavior relative to control, regulation, and coordination of machines and man. Information theory plays an essential part in this field because it deals with a set of possibilities. Relevant information about the situation increases the probability that an effective decision about a course of action will be made. Nurses gather information about the patient, family, and environment through communication, observation, and types of relationships established. They make inferences and decisions for nursing intervention on the basis of the information. This approach to the study of health care systems offers a method for the scientific treatment of the complex system in the real world of nursing practice.

Analysis of nursing situations suggests that patients are not always consciously aware of their health problems, and that the conditions for perceiving events are not present; for example, in a situation in which there is inadequate information about what is planned for the patient. When the conditions are unknown to the patient, a barrier makes action difficult, if not impossible. Communication is, therefore, an important aspect of the nurse-patient relationship.

---

[12] Daniel Howland, "A Hospital System Model," *Nursing Research*, Fall 1963, pp. 232-236.

Communication—One Facet of Interpersonal Relations

The chief function of language in society is to facilitate cooperation and interaction among individuals. A significant factor in man's cultural growth was his gradual development of language.

Language is so much a part of one's daily life that it is taken for granted. Through language persons pass on experiences and thoughts to each succeeding generation. Although words are the symbols of man's thinking, they provide a certain difficulty akin to the difference in perception of reality. Words have different meaning for different persons. The experience of the listener, speaker, or reader determines the full effect of the meaning of words.

Communication is an interchange of thoughts and opinions among individuals. Verbal communication is effective when it satisfies basic desires for recognition, participation, and self-realization by direct personal contact between persons. Nonverbal communication includes gestures, facial expressions, actions, and postures of listening and feeling. Communication is the means whereby social interaction and learning take place. An individual who is unable to speak with ease, clarity, and assurance, and who is unable to listen with comprehension and assimilation, may have difficulty with social adaptation. To be effective, communication must take place in an atmosphere of mutual respect and desire for understanding. Communication is affected by the interrelationships of an individual's goal, needs, and expectations; thus, the environmental situation has a social and personal dimension.

Each profession has developed its own language and assumes that the listener—for example, a patient—understands the meaning of the words. In order for health professionals to communicate health information, it is essential that they use language that has meaning for the public and that can be understood within its frame of reference.[13]

Meyer[14] attempted to determine the effects of communication

13 Surgeon General's Conference on Health Communication, November 1962, U.S. Department of Health, Education, and Welfare, U.S. Government Printing Office, Washington, D.C., February, 1963.

14 Mary E. Meyers, "The Effect of Types of Communication on the Patient's Reaction to Stress," *Nursing Research*, Spring 1964, pp. 126-131.

on patient care. Findings of the study indicated that in order to minimize or reduce tension in nursing situations, patients must receive specific information to give meaning to what is happening to them. Information gives the patient a means for cognitive structuring of impending events. "If a measure of the stress a patient feels upon hospitalization is related to the deprivation he experiences, then it follows that the communication approach will negate or at least minimize some of the stress inherent in hospitalization." If nurses are concerned with patient-centered care and continue to explore the psychosocial aspects of care, structured oral and written communication that can be understood by patients is one approach suggested.[15]

Nurses in performing their functions in a specific type of environment have opportunities to study interaction in concrete situations. Nurses are constantly observing individuals who are experiencing stress, fear, and anxiety, as well as joy and happiness. They are constantly observing individuals' response to pain, to various types of illness, and to different kinds of therapy. Nurses gather information about an individual's reaction to his environment. Skills in interviewing are essential, too, for nurses to assess needs and perceptions of patients. Communication, which is related to perception and is a critical variable in studying interpersonal relationships, is a way of systematically assessing how an individual views a particular situation and forms relationships. Another approach would be to observe the behavior of individuals for cues that indicate characteristics of patterns of patient reactions to nurses actions. The basic elements in the dynamics of nursing can be viewed in the context of human relationships in complex environmental situations.

The effects of one's perception influence communication and interpersonal relationships with other individuals. Nurses are concerned with their own actions and those of others. The basic elements of action lead one to know what an individual can do, what he is trying to do, and what he intends to do about his health problem. What is perceived by individuals may be judged by them as favorable or unfavorable. Nurses influence the

[15] Mary F. Bucklin Mohammed, "Patients' Understanding of Written Health Information," *Nursing Research*, Spring 1964, pp. 100-108.

patient's perception, communication, and relations, and either motivate him to action or prevent him from action.

Summary

The dynamics of nursing can be described as a constant restructuring of relationships between the nurse and patient to cope with existential problems and to learn ways of adapting or adjusting to changes in daily activities. A basic element of analysis, the nursing act, as a sequence of behaviors in the nursing process, was presented. The concepts of perception and interpersonal relations are dynamic dimensions of the nursing process. Verbal and nonverbal communications are a facet of the process. There are implications that the perception of persons as they establish interpersonal relationships with individuals and groups in various social systems influences the means to achieve a goal of optimum health for each person.

The components of nursing were distinguished by the processes involved and showed nursing as a dynamic system related to other systems. The processes referred to were those of communicating, relating, using knowledge, gathering information, making decisions, and evaluating consequences of decisions. These processes refer to operations associated with human behavior in nursing situations, with knowledge, and its utilization in specific situations.

A quest for usable information furnishes a common ground on which the nurse practitioner, the teacher, and the researcher can meet. Communication and collaboration among nurses will improve theory through testing it in the real world of practice and will improve practice through the utilization of theoretical evidence.

Selected Readings

American Nurses' Association, "ANA Board Approves a Definition of Nursin Practice," *American Journal of Nursing*, December 1955, p. 1474.

American Nurses' Association, "The Biennial," *American Journal of Nursing* November 1946, pp. 728-746.

American Nurses' Association, "Professional Nursing Defined," *America Journal of Nursing*, May 1937, p. 518.

Amidon, Edmund, and Hough, John B. (eds.), *Interaction Analysis: Theory Research and Application*, Addison-Wesley, Reading, Mass., 1967.

Bales, R. F., *Interaction Process Analysis*, Addison-Wesley, Cambridge, Mass 1950.

Berelson, Bernard, *The Behavioral Sciences Today*, Basic Books, New York 1963.

Berelson, Bernard, and Steiner, G. A. *Human Behavior: An Inventory o Scientific Findings*, Harcourt Brace, New York, 1964.

Bloom, Benjamin, *Stability and Change in Human Characteristics*, John Wiley and Sons, New York, 1964.

Brown, Esther L., *Nursing for the Future*, Russell Sage Foundation, New York, 1948, p. 73.

Combs, Arthur W., and Snygg, Donald, *Individual Behavior: A Perceptua Approach to Behavior*, rev. ed., Harper and Brothers, New York, 1959

Conant, Lucy H., "Use of Bales Interaction Process Analysis to Study Nurse Patient Interaction," *Nursing Research*, Fall 1965, pp. 304-309.

Diers, Donna, and Leonard, Robert C., "Interaction Analysis in Nursin Research," *Nursing Research*, Summer 1966, pp. 225-228.

Dodge, Joan, "Nurse-Doctor Relations and Attitudes Toward the Patient, *Nursing Research*, 1960, pp. 32-38.

Folta, Jeannette R., "The Perception of Death," *Nursing Research*, Summe 1965, pp. 232-235.

Fromm, Erich, *The Art of Loving*, Bantam Books, New York, 1963.

Goldiamond, I., "Perception," in A. J. Bachrach, *The Experimental Foundations of Clinical Psychology*, 1962, pp. 280-340.

Gowan, Naomi, and Morris, Miriam, "Nurses Responses to Expressed Patient Needs," *Nursing Research*, Winter 1964, pp. 68-78.

Hammond, Kenneth R., "Clinical Inference in Nursing, II. A Psychologist's Viewpoint," *Nursing Research*, Winter 1966, pp. 27-38.

Hammond, Kenneth R. et al., "Clinical Inference in Nursing Analyzing Cognitive Tasks Representative of Nursing Problems," *Nursing Research*, Spring 1966, pp. 134-138.

Hayes, Joyce, and Larson, Kenneth, *Interacting with Patients: Communications for General and Psychiatric Nurses*, Macmillan, New York, 1963.

Henderson, Virginia, *The Nature of Nursing*, Macmillan, New York, 1966.

Huxley, A. L., *The Doors of Perception*, Harper and Brothers, New York, 1954.

Jenkins, C. D., "Group Differences in Perception: A Study of Community Beliefs and Feelings About Tuberculosis," *American Journal of Sociology*, January 1966.

Jones, Marshall (ed.), *The Nebraska Symposium on Motivation*, Lincoln, Nebraska, University of Nebraska Press, 1955, H. Murray, "Toward a Classification of Interaction," p. 252.

Kelly, Katherine, "Clinical Inference in Nursing, I. A Nurse's Viewpoint," *Nursing Research*, Winter 1966, pp. 23-26.

Kelly, Katherine J., and Hammond, Kenneth R., "An Approach to the Study of Clinical Inference in Nursing, Part I., Part II, Part III.," *Nursing Research*, Fall 1964, pp. 314-322.

Kogan, Kate L., and Jackson, Joan, "Role Perception in Hospital Interaction," *Nursing Research*, Spring 1956, pp. 75-79.

Kumata H., and Schramm, W., "A Pilot Study of Cross-Cultural Meaning," *Public Opinion Quarterly*, 1956.

National Education Association Yearbook, *Perceiving, Behaving, Becoming: A New Focus for Education*, Association in Supervision and Curriculum Development, 1962.

Parsons, Talcott, and Shils, E. (eds.), *Toward a General Theory of Action*, Harvard University Press, Cambridge, Mass., 1952.

Phenix, Philip H., *Realms of Meaning*, McGraw-Hill, New York, 1966.

Rawlinson, May E., "Projection in Relation to Interpersonal Perception," *Nursing Research*, Spring 1965, pp. 114-118.

Rogers, Carl, and Rothelsberger, F. J., "Barriers and Gateways to Communication," *Harvard Business Review*, 1952, pp. 28-34.

Roy, S. N., *Some Aspects of Multivariate Analysis*, John Wiley and Sons, New York, 1957.

Schultz, W. C., *FIRO: A Three-dimensional Theory of Interpersonal Behavior*, Holt Rinehart & Winston, New York, 1960.

Suppes, P., and Atkinson, R. C., *Learning Models for Multiperson Interaction*, Stanford University Press, Palo Alto, Calif., 1960.

Taguiri, Renato, and Luigi, Petrullo (eds.), *Person, Perception and Interpersonal Behavior*, Standford University Press, Palo Alto, Calif., 1958.

Thomas, Lawrence G., "Implications of Transaction Theory," *The Educational Forum*, January 1968, pp. 145-155.

Winn, Ralph (ed.), *Transaction Theory and Perception*, Philosophical Library, New York, 1959.

Chapter 7

The Problem in Retrospect

Reflections on Changes in Society and Nursing

The discoveries of science have altered the world around us. A mere glimpse of the effects of the accumulation, retrieval, and dissemination of information through automation and computers bears witness to this fact. Factors such as mass media of communication, mechanization, urbanization, increased life expectancy, and social and geographic mobility have brought about changes in the attitudes and customs of individuals, and changes in community life in general. Innovations in transportation and communication, the basic avenues of social interaction, have brought the people of the world closer together.

The simple act of nurturing in ancient civilizations, extended in time and place to the present, appears as an aggregate of health services. Nurses comprise one of the largest health groups in the United States. They have become essential human resources for the delivery of health services by social organizations. They provide a special service to help meet individual and group needs in coping with health, illness, and death. This service consists of health teaching, health maintenance, and health restoration.

Historically nursing has two roots, both of which emanated

from the basic needs of man in society. The first was man's need to survive. Disease, injury, wars, epidemics, and disasters have always been a threat to life. Nursing was conceived as a helping profession. Nurses provided care for the sick, injured, and infirm. As knowledge was discovered and used to control some diseases and to prevent some epidemics and disasters, the responsibilities assumed by nurses expanded from primarily care of the sick to include prevention of disease as well as promotion and restoration of health.

The second historical root of nursing was man's need for help as an individual. Human beings have always exhibited similarities in basic needs such as feeding, grooming, learning, and so forth, and they have responded to care at times when these needs were met by someone other than themselves or a member of the family.

Modern organized nursing has emphasized the individual, the group, and the environment as major components in its field of practice. Changes in society and in knowledge available for use have caused nurses to question their practice and to seek opportunities for continuing education.

Notes on Social and Educational Change in the United States

The social and health legislation of the late 1960's has reiterated the value of the human being in society, and has placed health and welfare high on the American scale of values. Explosive advances in science and technology have led to rapid change in health care systems. Yet, the basic structure and functions of social organizations responsible for the delivery of health services have not altered appreciably the means by which knowledge is utilized for expanding roles, functions, and new responsibilities.

Occupation patterns have produced kaleidoscopic functions. Increased technology has brought about increased specialization. Brainpower is replacing manpower. Research has become a definite and permanent national characteristic. As a result of man's progress through research, the economic structure of the

United States that affects living standards has been modified during the past few decades. In the past, the basic needs for living —food, clothing, housing—were the dominant economic problems for the majority of citizens. Today, there is a shift in the economy to the need for services of many types, such as health, education, and recreation. Moreover, financial support of these services is a new economic problem.

Evidence points to a changing American population—to a country of older persons. The family unit in America has been altered. What was considered an extended kinship group in the early part of the century has almost disappeared in American society. The nuclear family, which consists of parents and children, is the most prevalent unit today. Values and norms of children differ from those of their parents. In a previous era, parents interpreted the world to the child, but the situation is often reversed today as the child interprets the world to his parents. The position of the elderly in the family structure varies from culture to culture, as does the position of youth.

Changes in society continue to have an impact on the educational system. Investment in educational opportunities for all Americans is considered intellectual capital that adds to the collective wealth of the nation. Two educational movements that have been gaining momentum in the past decade have been the expansion of community colleges and the emphasis on continuing education for adults. Community colleges have broadened their functions to meet some of the educational, cultural, and recreational needs of the people in the communities they serve. Continuing education programs for adults have begun to offer the opportunity for individuals to avail themselves of a variety of learning experiences that not only are vocational in nature, but also provide for liberal education, and cultural and recreational diversions. As new knowledge is disseminated and automation takes over in some industries, retraining of manpower becomes essential. Twenty-five years ago a secondary education was a goal of the majority of individuals. The question today is "Who should go to which college?"

A highly technological society such as the United States demands an educated citizenry. Human resources constitute a democratic nation's primary source of power and must not be left to develop by chance. The complexity of modern society makes extraordinarily heavy demands on the intelligence and understanding of all people. Americans look to the schools to prepare citizens for leadership; for useful, happy living; for a world of work; and for preservation of a free society. The demand for post-high-school education by the future voters as well as continued education for adults indicates some change in attitudes toward education.

Increased specialization, technologic changes, social, occupational, and geographic mobility, increased leisure time, a population of college-bound youth, and the demand for more health workers have challenged the educational programs and the work situations for nurses. Changes in the social and educational spheres of living have brought about an increase in health care systems, an awareness of the need for continuous learning for professionals, and the institutionalization of health care. Health practices and medical and nursing services exist to meet a social need, and are inextricably bound to all the movements and change that affect man in society.

Factors That Influenced Changes in Nursing

The population increase, increased life expectancy, and the expansion of health facilities and services have influenced some changes in nursing. Movement from private duty nursing to one of employment by agencies has changed some of the functions of nurses. Moreover, a technological society in which specialization has been increasing in direct proportion to the knowledge explosion has called for specialized kinds of nursing care. Furthermore, a college-bound population of high school graduates has influenced changes in nursing education.

In the United States the majority of practitioners a half century ago were engaged in private duty nursing. With an increase in population came the expansion of health facilities and services. The Hill-Burton Act of 1946, which provided grants for construction, has become synonymous with hospital building programs. The expansion of these institutions created a demand for more nursing personnel. The extension of the Hill-Burton legislation will continue to spiral this need.[1]

Paralleling the increase in hospital beds in the 1940's and 1950's was the employment of more nurses by hospitals. Today, the majority of nurses are employed by hospitals.[2] The introduction of nonprofessional personnel in the field of nursing practice, particularly in hospitals and nursing homes, has greatly increased since the 1950's.[3]

Voluntary health insurance programs offered a way to resolve some of the financial problems of the hospital as well as those of the patients. The growth of medical care insurance has been related to an increase in the numbers of individuals using hospital facilities. The passage of Public Law 89-97 commonly referred to as Medicare[4] has continued to influence the demand for nursing personnel.

Specialization in medical practice has influenced nursing practice. A case in point is the current demand for nurses with specialized knowledge, ability, and skills to provide nursing care and emergency life-saving care for patients admitted to coronary care units in hospitals. Short, intensive training programs have been established throughout the country to retrain nurses for these specific technologic functions. The complementary and collaborative relationships between nurses and physicians in these units demonstrate daily that they function from a similar frame of reference from which to make split-second decisions to use their knowledge to assist individuals maintain life. Demands are made, too, for nurses with specialized knowledge and skills to provide care for patients in need of renal dialysis, for patients with neurological problems, etc.

As physicians became more specialized, they delegated some of their activities to nurses, and nurses accepted this responsibility. Concomitant with the assignment of technical functions from physicians to nurses was the delegation to the nurse aides and

[1] United States Department of Health, Education, and Welfare, *The Hill-Harris Amendments of 1964,* Reprint, HEW Indicators, September 1964.

[2] American Nurses' Association, *Facts About Nursing,* American Nurses' Association, New York, 1969, p. 10.

[3] Ibid., pp. 20, 24.

[4] Social Security Amendments of 1965, Health Insurance for the Aged Act.

practical (vocational) nurses of tasks once performed only by "registered professional nurses."

An essential part of any profession is a nucleus of scientists. One recent change in the nursing profession has been the increase in the number of nurses seeking research preparation at the doctoral level. Any profession that has as its primary mission the delivery of social services requires continuous research to discover new knowledge that can be applied to improve practice.

Behavioral scientists have found in nursing a fertile field for testing their theories. Study after study has been reported about the role of nurses and organizations in which nurses perform various roles and responsibilities. Although the findings of these studies cannot be generalized to the total nurse population, some clues are provided that have implications for reassessing nursing functions and responsibilities. Reismann and Rohrer's[5] study, for example, shows discrepancies between what nurses verbalize as their role and functions, and what the researchers' observations of the functions of these nurses actually indicate. Nurses in this study described their functions as those for which the educational programs had prepared them—to give direct patient care—while in fact they were expected to perform in managerial roles.

In the introduction to a book of readings, Mauksch[6] notes that:

. . . the nurse is the one functionary of the hospital who is at the patient care unit continuously. All others, including the physician, come and go. . . . The nurse must understand the principles of organization and administration because, in reality, whether she likes it or not, she has become *de facto* administrator in the complexity of patient care.

Although some of the studies in nursing indicate that nurses function in a managerial role, some of the trends show that a few innovations are occurring to change the focus of some of the management functions. Changes in medical practice and in patterns of health care, such as extended care facilities, and technologic advances have prompted some nurses to reassess their

5 Leonard Reismann and John H. Rohrer (eds.), *Change and Dilemma in the Nursing Profession*, G. P. Putnam & Sons, New York, 1957.

6 James K. Skipper Jr. and Robert C. Leonard, *Social Interaction and Patient Care*, J. B. Lippincott, Philadelphia, 1965, p. xiii.

roles and responsibilities and to focus on the management of patient care rather than hospitals wards.

Some studies have been conducted and some are ongoing that attempt to define the role, functions, and responsibilities of the clinical specialist in nursing.[7, 8, 9, 10] These studies have used different methods, but they all seek to determine roles, responsibilities, and to the use of knowledge by nurses to perform activities that are distinctively nursing. The role of the clinical specialist that is emerging brings the nurse back to patient care, the purpose for which many individuals entered the profession initially. Some nurses functioning as clinical specialists have demonstrated a change in their practice from an intuitive and empirical approach to a humanistic and scientific approach, using knowledge to plan, implement, and evaluate nursing care.

The basis for the practice of nursing is knowledge; its activity is guided by the intellect, and its intellectual activity is applied in the practical realm. The primary mission of social service oriented professions is to deliver a specific kind of service based on knowledge. Professionals from various fields of study may have a similar background of knowledge to assist individuals adapt to changing health states. **A distinguishing characteristic among professionals, however, is the way in which they use knowledge to perform particular activities.**

Communication of knowledge and the application of knowledge in the practice of nursing in the real world are essential components of the educational programs for nursing. Research, teaching, and practice are three elements in a profession that are interrelated and complementary. If nurses are to understand and participate in the role demanded of them in today's world and tomorrow's, means must be found to close the gap between the

7 Laura Simms, "The Clinical Nursing Specialist: An Experiment," *Nursing Outlook,* August 1964, pp. 26-28.

8 Doris Carnevali and Little, Dolores, "Tuberculosis Patients and the Nurse," *Nursing Outlook,* May 1965, pp. 78-80.

9 National League for Nursing, *Blueprint for Action in Hospital Nursing,* Clinical Specialist, 1964, pp. 85-98.

10 Frances Reiter, "The Nurse Clinician," *American Journal of Nursing,* February 1966, pp. 274-280.

discovery of knowledge, communication of that knowledge, and its application to nursing practice.

The teachers in the basic education programs prepare students to enter the field as beginning practitioners. Employers, however, often utilize these beginning practitioners as managers of patient care units. The nonprofessional nursing personnel have assumed the role of giving direct care to patients, and the nurses have been required to supervise them in this role. This is one of the changes that must be scrutinized by members of the profession as they make decisions for the future. A brief review of some of the modifications in nursing education for nursing practice indicates that changes have been recommended in each decade for the past fifty years, although the suggestions have not always been acted upon and implemented by the profession.

Changes in Education for Nursing Practice

Placing nursing education within the general system of education is not a new idea in this country. Discussions of university education for nurses began at the turn of the century. The following examples put the direction of nursing education in historical perspective.

In 1903, a statement appeared that "engineers must be educated by engineers, surgeons by surgeons, and nurses by nurses—each profession in its own school, under its own separate faculty, and controlled only by the university."[11] A few years later Beard[12] wrote that "the university education for nurses, as a department of instruction, is an accomplished fact."

A review of the guides for curriculum development for schools of nursing indicates changes in each of three decades. In 1917, the Committee on Education of the National League for Nursing Education made one of the first attempts to guide schools

[11] Doctor Worcester, "The Education of Nurses," *The University Record* Chicago, Illinois, May 1903, p. 1. Quoted from U.S. Bureau of Education Bulletin No. 7, 1912.

[12] Richard Olding Beard, "The University Education of the Nurse," *Teachers College Record*, May 1910, pp. 27-40.

in setting standards for nursing education.[13] The study of social sciences was suggested as part of the curriculum. Ten years later the committee identified the functions and responsibilities of the nurse.[14] The case study method was recommended as a tool for learning nursing and social and health concepts and qualities of leadership were mentioned as areas to be developed in the curriculum. The 1937 guide[15] presented the profession with concepts such as critical thinking, individual differences, motivation for continued professional growth, and principles of learning.

Bixler[16] analyzed the professional status of nursing in 1945, then reexamined it in 1959, using identical criteria, to determine the progress made toward meeting the criteria for a profession. One major problem that continued to present itself in 1959 was the lack of an organized body of knowledge and its utilization in nursing situations. The problem has not yet been resolved.

Studies have been reported for years describing education for the profession. The Ginzberg[17] and Brown[18] reports brought into sharp focus some of the problems facing nursing and nurses. A study at midcentury presented a classification of schools (data collected from 97 percent of all schools) and indicated a need for redefining objectives and standards.[19] The period of the 1950's saw a reassessment of nursing as a profession. Establishment of the National Accrediting Service within the National League for Nursing has influenced changes in nursing education.

[13] Committee on Education of the National League for Nursing Education, *Standard Curriculum for Schools of Nursing*, The Waverly Press, Baltimore, 1917.

[14] Committee on Education of the National League for Nursing Education, *A Curriculum for Schools of Nursing*, sixth ed. rev. NLNE, New York, 1927.

[15] Committee on Curriculum of the National League for Nursing Education, *A Curriculum Guide for Schools of Nursing*, 2nd rev., NLNE, New York, 1937.

[16] Genevieve Bixler, "Professional Status of Nursing," *American Journal of Nursing*, August 1959, pp. 1142-1147.

[17] Eli Ginzberg, *Committee on the Function of Nursing Services, A Program for the Nursing Profession*, Macmillan, New York, 1949.

[18] Esther L. Brown, *Nursing for the Future*, Russell Sage Foundation, New York, 1948.

[19] National Committee for Improvement of Nursing, Margaret West and Christy Hawkins, *Nursing Schools at the Mid-Century*, New York, 1950.

In 1955, representatives of the Council of Member Agencies
of the Department of Baccalaureate and Higher Degree Programs
of the National League for Nursing recommended a redefinition
of baccalaureate and higher education for nursing; changes in
curriculums were to become effective by 1963.[20] Up to 1963, the
undergraduate programs offered curriculums leading to specialization in teaching, administration and public health nursing. Since
1963, all accredited undergraduate programs offering a major
in nursing have provided basic education to prepare the professional practitioner. Graduate education was defined as programs of study that prepared nurses for specialization in an area
of clinical nursing.

In 1951, a small book was published that influenced a major
change in education for nursing. This tiny volume[21] proposed a
plan for educating the bedside nurse within the educational
institution called the junior-community college. It went on to
suggest graduate education for the teachers and administrators
of these programs. The ideas were tested in selected institutions
in several regions of the country during a five-year "Cooperative
Research Project." At the completion of the project, an evaluation
of the experimental programs and of the graduates was published
in a final report.[22] This project identified technical as opposed to
professional education for nursing. In addition, it highlighted
the necessity for a study of baccalaureate programs to determine
the differentiating characteristics between technical and professional education for nursing.

The biennial convention of the American Nurses' Association[23]
in 1966 will be recorded in history as a milestone in recommenda-
tions for change in the education of nurses for the future. The
House of Delegates of this organization voted to support the

[20] National League for Nursing, Department of Baccalaureate and Higher
Degree Programs, Council of Member Agencies, Minutes of the 1955 meeting,
New York, 1955.

[21] Mildred L. Montag, *The Education of Nursing Technicians,* G. P. Putnam's Sons, New York, 1951.

[22] Mildred L. Montag, *Community College Education for Nursing,* Mc-
Graw-Hill, New York, 1959.

[23] American Nurses' Association, *Proceedings of the 1966 Biennial Convention,* New York, 1966.

position[24] that professional nurses of the future be prepared in institutions of higher education in the baccalaureate programs, and that technical education for nursing be offered in junior-community colleges. Recent data have indicated trends in the direction proposed by the American Nurses' Association position paper.

Nursing students are being educated in three different types of formal basic programs. Two of these are administered within the general system of education: (1) the bachelor of science in nursing, administered within colleges and universities; and (2) the associate degree nursing program, administered within the junior-community colleges. A third program is conducted by hospitals and leads to a diploma. The graduates of these three types of programs (of four to five years, and two years to three years in length respectively) are required to pass the same state licensing examination to become "registered professional nurses."

The three basic programs differ in administration and control, in the objectives to be achieved by the students upon graduation, in faculty qualifications and responsibilities, and in the student population. One characteristic common to all three types of programs is that upon graduation and successful achievement in the state licensing examination, all graduates hold the legal title "registered professional nurse." This indicates that by state law they have met the minimum requirements of the law and should be able to plan and administer safe patient care. An inference is made that graduates who pass the same licensing examination had some common learning experiences. Yet, it is loudly proclaimed by some nurses that there are real differences among the three programs. Another inference is made that if there are three different types of educational programs, there are different levels of nursing practice. Some employers, however, consider all the graduates in the same category of personnel, the "registered professional nurse" (R.N.). The differences in the kind and quality of nursing care given by these graduates have not been described clearly by the profession.

A fourth program in the United States prepares the vocational

[24] American Nurses' Association, "ANA Position Paper on Nursing Education," *American Journal of Nursing,* December 1965, pp. 106-111.

(practical) nurse. If one makes some random observations in hospitals, the graduates of all four programs may be performing similar tasks for patients. Similarities and differences in the expected performance of graduates of these several programs may be clear in the minds of some individuals in nursing, but they have not been tested widely, nor communicated clearly to the employers, the physicians, the paramedical groups, and the public.

Nursing action depends on decision, and decision depends on knowledge and communication skills. Nursing action by the professional, technical, and vocational nurse will vary in proportion to variations in decisions made by each in nursing situations. These variations in decisions are directly associated with differences in knowledge of the natural and behavioral sciences, and in communication and interpersonal skills used by the professional, the technical, and the vocational nurse.

Education for nursing practice is in a period of change, probably the first real change since the implementation of the Nightingale system at the turn of the century and the beginning of the education of nurse technicians in the community college in the 1950's and 1960's. Nightingale[25] probably initiated the first revolution in nursing education and nursing practice in 1890. Peplau,[26] however, was probably one of the first nurses to formulate a precise definition of nursing from which a set of concepts were derived that form the foundation for "psychodynamic nursing." Her ideas provide a theoretical frame of reference for nursing. Rogers[27] has brought the second revolution in nursing into sharp focus.

Reflections on changes in nursing in society have raised a fundamental question: *Have the basic responsibilities of nurses really changed in the past twenty-five to fifty years? What essential characteristics have continued to be a part of nursing over time?*

25 Florence Nightingale, *Notes on Nursing: What It Is and What It Is Not*, Facsimile of the First Edition printed in London, J. B. Lippincott, Philadelphia, 1959.

26 Hildegard E. Peplau, *Interpersonal Relations in Nursing*, G. P. Putman's Sons, New York, 1952.

27 Martha E. Rogers, *Educational Revolution in Nursing*, Macmillan, New York, 1961.

Characteristics That Persist Within the Changes

Transitory changes have permeated nursing, but a few basic elements have continuously remained an integral part of nursing practice. *Nursing continues to be a helping profession. Nurses provide a service that meets a social need. A part of this service is to give care to individuals and groups who are acutely and moderately ill and usually hospitalized.* Nurses give care to those individuals who have a chronic disease and those who need rehabilitation to help them use their potential ability to function as human beings. Nurses offer guidance and counseling for individuals and groups to help them maintain health. Nurses are partners with physicians in promoting health, in preventing disease, and in managing patient care. They cooperate and collaborate with physicians, families, and paramedical groups to coordinate a plan of health care for individuals and groups. Nurses are being recognized as the key figures in the delivery of health services today.

A part of the service provided by nurses deals with specific technical skills that they are expected to possess. Two such skills, observation and communication, are important methods for collecting information to make decisions to implement a plan for nursing care. Some technical skills, commonly referred to as "procedures," *have been and continue to be an essential aspect of nursing, such as accurate measurement of blood pressure, pulse, temperature, and respiration.* These skills are important for gathering reliable and valid data about some of the physiological parameters of individuals' health states. Skills necessary for implementing physician-initiated therapy, such as intubation, inhalation, and drainage of body cavities, have been a part of the nurses' repertoire for years. Some technological changes have required that nurses learn additional skills for specific situations, such as monitoring physiologic parameters of patients in specialized care units in hospitals, care of premature infants, and health guidance in nurse clinics, and health agencies, and homes.

Some of the technical skills involved in caring for patients in hospitals have been delegated to nonprofessional nursing personnel. Thus, **in seeking to identify differentiating characteristics of** professional nurses one must look to the uncommon knowledge, skills, and set of preferences that differ from those outside the group and to the legal right to perform specific functions. Many persons, for example, can count pulse and respiratory rates, take a blood pressure, or give a hypodermic injection. These skills are common. Professionals, however, use the information attained from the performance of these techniques to plan a course of action to maintain internal and external equilibrium in patients. They evaluate the information against their knowledge to determine changes in these phenomena in a patient, and then to determine whether or not these changes are significant and related to the person's health state.

Some of the functions of nurses have not changed; some of the tasks have been delegated to nonprofessional personnel while nurses have assumed physician-delegated activities and hospital management activities. The knowledge available for use in deciding courses of nursing action has increased. Nurses are expected to synthesize knowledge from natural and behavioral sciences, and to use knowledge in making decisions to meet basic needs of individuals that are immediate in a nursing situation, and also, to plan with individuals to help them learn ways to cope with illness and health problems in the future, and to adapt to changes in health.

Theory development for nursing is essential if professional nurses are to continue to assume their roles and responsibilities in an ever changing society. Theoretical models organize sets of concepts that are related and provide methodology for gathering information that is essential for decision making in nursing. Theories offer explanations of behaviors of individuals in particular situations. Theories provide a framework for organization of phenomena and for studying the elements that interact with each other and are related.

The theoretical frame of reference presented in this book has been derived from basic elements in nursing that have and will continue to persist over time. Man, the human organism, is the central focus for the framework. His adaptation to life and health is influenced by internal and external environmental factors.

Summary

The social and educational changes affecting man in society have influenced changes in the educational programs and the work situations for nurses. This chapter discussed some of the basic elements that have continued to remain a part of nursing over time.

Nursing as a bio-psycho-social phenomenon has as its focus man, social interaction, and social movements. Some understanding of man and his environment is prerequisite to understanding the nature of nursing. Today, it is essential that nurses be educated for change; that they understand what it means for individuals to change their patterns of living to adapt to health states; that they be perceptive of the social environment, the physical, emotional, and intellectual needs of man; and that they be flexible in coping with them.

The intellectual base for nursing of necessity includes some conceptualization of the process of application of knowledge in the practice of the profession. This chapter has highlighted some of the changes in society and in nursing.

Selected Readings

Brown, Mary Louise, "Highlights of the Occupational Health Nursing Study," *American Association of Industrial Nurses Journal*, May 1965.

Davis, Fred (ed.), *The Nursing Profession*, John Wiley and Sons, New York, 1966.

Department of the Interior, Bureau of Education, *Biennial Survey of Education 1916-1918*, Volume IV., Chapter 6, "Nurse Training Schools, 1917-1918," U.S. Government Printing Office, Washington, D.C., 1921, pp. 549-646.

Duvall, Evelyn, *Family Development*, 2nd ed., J. B. Lippincott, Philadelphia, 1962.

Galbraith, John K., *The Affluent Society*, Houghton Mifflin, Boston, 1958.

Jensen, Gale, Liverright, A. A., and Hallenbach, Wilbur (eds.), *Adult Education: Outlines of an Emerging Field of University Study*, Adult Education Association, 1964.

Johnstone, John W. C., and Rivera, Ramon J., *Volunteers for Learning*, Aldine Publishing Co., Chicago, Ill., 1965.

Journal of the American Academy of Arts and Sciences, *Daedalus*, "Toward the Year 2,000, Work in Progress," Summer 1967.

Journal of the American Academy of Arts and Sciences, *Daedalus*, "Conditions of World Order," Spring 1966.

Journal of the American Academy of Arts and Sciences, *Daedalus*, "Science and Culture," Winter 1965.

Kluckholm, Florence, and Strodtbeck, Fred, *Variations in Value Orientation*, Row and Peterson, Evanston, Ill., 1961.

Lambertsen, Eleanor, *Education for Nursing Leadership*, J. B. Lippincott, Philadelphia, 1958.

Linton, Ralph, *The Tree of Culture*, abridged by Adelin Linton, Vintage Books, New York, 1958.

Medeseker, Leland, *The Junior College: Progress and Prospect*, McGraw-Hill, New York. 1960.

Meyer, Genevieve R., "Conflict and Harmony in Nursing Values," *Nursing Outlook*, 1959, pp. 398-399.

Meyer, Genevieve R., *Tenderness and Technique, Nursing Values in Transition*, Institute of Industrial Relations, University of California, Los Angeles, 1959.

National Commission for the Study of Nursing and Nursing Education, *American Journal of Nursing*, February 1970, pp. 279-294.

Ninth Yearbook of the National Society for the Study of Education, Part II., "The Nurse in Education," University of Chicago Press, 1910, pp. 18-59.

President's Commission on Higher Education, Report to the President, *Higher Education for American Democracy: Establishing Goals*, Harper and Brothers, New York, 1948.

President's Committee on Education Beyond High School, Second Report to the President, U.S. Government Printing Office, Washington, D.C. 1957.

Russell, Charles, *Liberal Education and Nursing*, Institute of Higher Education, Bureau of Publications, Teachers College, Columbia University, New York, 1959.

Shock, Nathan (ed.), *Aging Around the World*, International Association of Gerontology, Fifth Congress in San Francisco, 1960, 4 Volumes, Columbia University Press, New York, 1962.

Shock, Nathan (ed.), *Some Social and Biological Aspects of Aging*, American Association for Advancement of Science, Washington, D.C., 1960.

Western Interstate Commission on Higher Education, *Nursing Education for Today, Tomorrow, the Day after That*, Proceedings of the First Annual Conference, March 1958, Boulder, Colorado, June 1958.

Chapter 8

Conclusion

This book has discussed some of the fundamental dimensions relevant for nursing. There are doubtless other phenomena of equal importance that have been omitted or treated tangentially. The purpose, as stated in the beginning, was to develop a conceptual frame of reference that has implications for practice, teaching, and research in nursing. Thus, multiple examples of nursing situations, techniques, and principles have not been treated specifically. The central focus discussed in the framework is man, the dynamic human organism, whose selected perceptions of objects, persons, and events influence his behavior, his social interaction, and his health. Nurses, as individuals, are an integral part of this framework. Nurses, as professionals, have roles to play at each stage of human growth and development to help human beings cope with health and illness.

The approach was guided by the conviction that although implicit theory is a part of practice, nursing is not yet a science. A personal concern of the author was to attempt to sort out of the past and present those factors that have consistently remained a part of nursing. Four word symbols—social systems, health, perception, and interpersonal relations—were selected and a few underlying concepts were developed. Concepts tell us what to observe and help nurses focus on selected aspects of reality. The set of concepts presented here will permit the description of nursing situations and behavioral processes. Continued exposition of a set of hypotheses may assist nurses in a process of inquiry into the nature of their practice and its relationship to human life and health.

The conceptual frame of reference presented in the previous chapters was formulated to serve several purposes. First, it is a way of thinking about the real world of nursing. This process of conceptualization revolves around several questions. What are the basic elements in nursing that have continued to remain an integral part of the field of practice over time? In what kind of settings are nurses employed? Are the current goals of nursing similar to those of the past few decades?

Second, it suggests an approach for selecting concepts perceived to be fundamental for the practice of professional nursing. *Third,* it shows a process for developing concepts that symbolize experiences within the physical, psychological, and social environment in nursing situations. The propositions are:

1. *Nursing is an observable behavior found in the health care systems in society.* Health care systems are social systems organized to attain or maintain health in people or restore them to health, or care of sick and dying.

   Nursing is an integral part of human life from conception to aging. A deduction from this assumption is that there are more similarities than differences in the adjectival varieties of nursing. Throughout the history of nursing and nursing education, nurses have been concerned exclusively with adjectives that describe the location of patients in hospitals, such as obstetric unit, pediatric unit, etc., and educators spend time selecting content for courses, for instance, in the field of medical-surgical nursing and pediatric nursing and saying that it differs substantially from each and every other kind of nursing. When one starts to compare the content of various courses in a nursing curriculum, the duplication and repetition is obvious. One of the differences is in the use of knowledge in caring for various age groups. The nursing process is observable as shown in this diagram.

Nurse $\rightarrow$ Perception $\leftrightarrow$ Judgment $\leftrightarrow$ Action

Reaction-Interaction-Transaction

Patient $\rightarrow$ Perception $\leftrightarrow$ Judgment $\leftrightarrow$ Action

Nurses infer the mental process of perception, judgment and action (Perception-Judgment-Action) from the reaction (verbal and nonverbal behavior) of nurse and patient to one another and to the environment. The interactions and transactions are observable since transactions result from a description of patterns of interaction.

2. *Nursing is a process of action, reaction, interaction and transaction between individuals and groups in social systems to achieve goals of health or adjustment to health problems.*

Perception is a fundamental concept in this process.

Perception = Function (Nurse $\leftrightharpoons$ Patient)

Perception = Function (Nurse $\leftrightharpoons$ Patient $\leftrightharpoons$ Physician)

Perception is the function of nurse and patient interactions.
Perception is the function of nurse and patient and physician interactions.

3. *The specific function of nursing is assistance to individuals to help them cope with a health problem or adjust to interference in their health state.*

The specific function of nursing is decision making and implementation of decisions for nursing intervention

Health = Function (Nurse $\leftrightharpoons$ Patient $\leftrightharpoons$ Physician $\leftrightharpoons$ Family $\leftrightharpoons$ Others)

Health is the function of nurse, patient, physician, family, and others interactions.

4. *The nurse works with individuals with a group referrent or with groups, not with individuals per se.*

The nurse helps individuals cope with their health state and changes in it when they cannot do this for themselves. The need for help may present itself at some particular time in the life cycle of man, from conception to aging, and in death. When the nurse is called on to help another person meet his basic needs to perform the activities of daily living, an interaction process occurs. Communication, verbal and nonverbal, is an essential factor in the establishment of interpersonal relationships. Initially, the relationship may be dyadic. As the client's needs are assessed, several individuals may enter into the relationship, such as the physician, the family, professional and nonprofessional persons. Thus a heterogeneous group, referred to as the health team, perform some functions that are distinct to each group. Some similar functions, such as health teaching, may overlap. The nurse appears to be a constant element in the patient's immediate environment and exerts some control of the decision-making process relative to the plan of care. This calls for a conscious awareness on the part of the nurse of the situational factors, such as physiologic deviations and social behaviors that may enhance or hinder the effectiveness of care. Therefore, the **perceptions** of the nurse, of the health client, of the physician, and of other professionals, **are critical elements in a nursing situation.**

The selective perceptions of both nurse and patient, resulting in actions, reactions, and interactions are influenced by situational variables. Some of these variables are the needs, goals, expectations, internal and external resources, and social class values of the interacting individuals. Therefore, some understanding of social systems within which individuals grow and develop appears essential if the goal to achieve a state of health feasible or appropriate for individuals and groups is to be attained. Moreover, the social organizations within which nurses function influence the means used to achieve goals. There are interacting forces in the life cycle of man at the level of the individuals, groups, and society. Processes, internal and external to the human organism, occurring in the life cycle, indicate the interrelationship of the concepts that make up the framework. Repetition here is essential to emphasize this point of interrelatedness. Generally speaking, an individual is born into his first social institution, the family. The family initiates the process of socialization through meeting the dependent needs of a baby and child. Communication and social interaction patterns are developed in this social system. The perceptual milieu of the child is bombarded with events, persons, and objects. As a child grows he begins to differentiate between persons and objects and learns ways to establish relationships in his social environment.

His knowledge is developed as his perceptual experiences are increased. The child is considered healthy if his development proceeds according to patterns of growth and behavior conceived to be those of the relatively normal individual in society. A concept of health includes a process of growth and development, and crises or interference, such as illness, may appear at any developmental phase of the life cycle.

Nursing, as a helping profession, is action oriented by virtue of the interpersonal process essential in determining the activities to be performed by nurses and patients. Actions, to be effective, imply knowledge and skills that are applicable in nursing situations.

The conceptual frame of reference presented in this book is abstract and deals with only a few elements of concrete situations. The four universal ideas, **social systems, health, perception,** and **interpersonal relations,** are relevant in every nursing situation.

If nurses are to assume the roles and responsibilities expected of them by employers, patients, physicians, and families (and, above all, if they are to fulfill their own expectations) the discovery of knowledge must be disseminated continuously to the practitioners in such a way that they are able to use it in their practice. One approach to this problem can be initiated in the educational program where the searching inquiry into the nature of nursing establishes the foundation for practice, for a way of thinking about practice, for continued learning, and for research.

Observations that are valid and reliable have been used in research in other fields of study over the years. Observations of human behavior are made daily by nurses in diverse settings. Descriptive data collected systematically provide cues for generating hypotheses for research in human behavior in nursing situations. Thus, information can be gathered and natural situations can be categorized as nurses systematically observe, record, analyze, and interpret behaviors of individuals in potentially stressful situations in their lives. Moreover, it would be impossible to design a plan for nursing care without the collection of relevant data. Nursing action without sufficient data for making decisions will be less than effective.

The main purpose of this book has been to present some ideas, suggestions, and speculations that may be helpful for students and teachers in building a conceptual frame of reference for analyzing some of the problems in nursing practice. This framework is offered for students, teachers, and practitioners to provide input from their experiences in concrete nursing situations. Although empirical knowledge exists, conceptual clarification will help nurses validate implicit theories through systematic experimentation. In nursing, perhaps more than in any other field, concepts and hypotheses are half formulated in what many nurses know intuitively. A systematic representation of nursing is required ultimately for developing a science to accompany a century or more of art in the everyday world of nursing.

> Without the Way
> There is no Going
> Without the Truth
> There is no Knowing
> Without the Life
> There is no Living.
>
> *Thomas ˋa Kempis*

Index